THE PICTURE BOOK OF

BIRDS

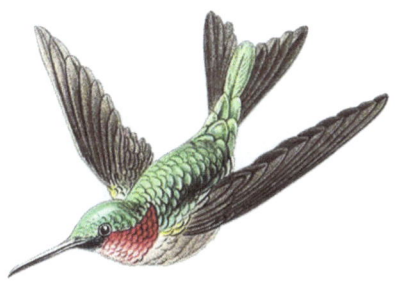

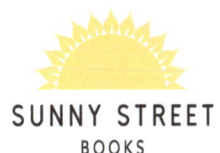

SUNNY STREET
BOOKS

BLUEBIRD

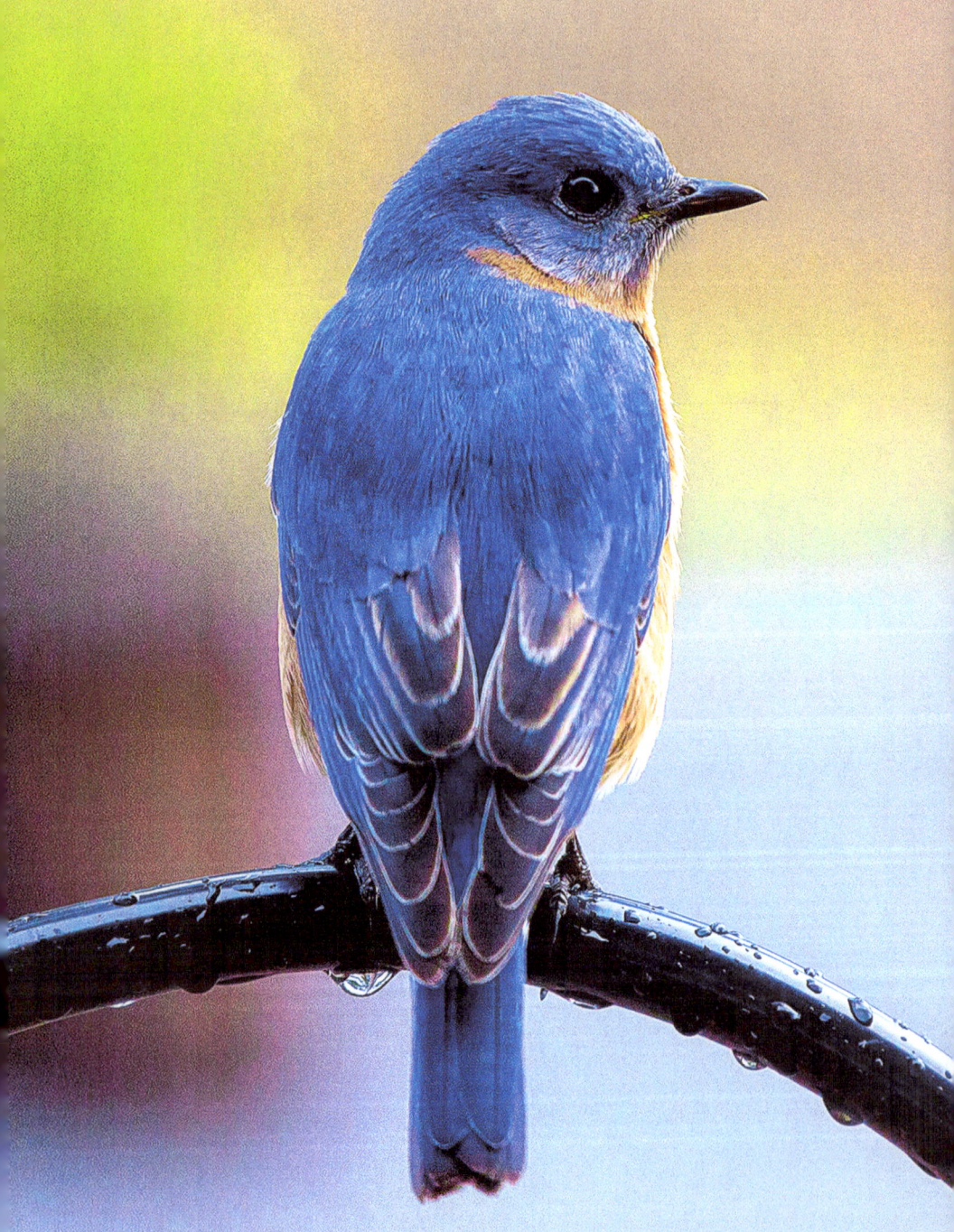

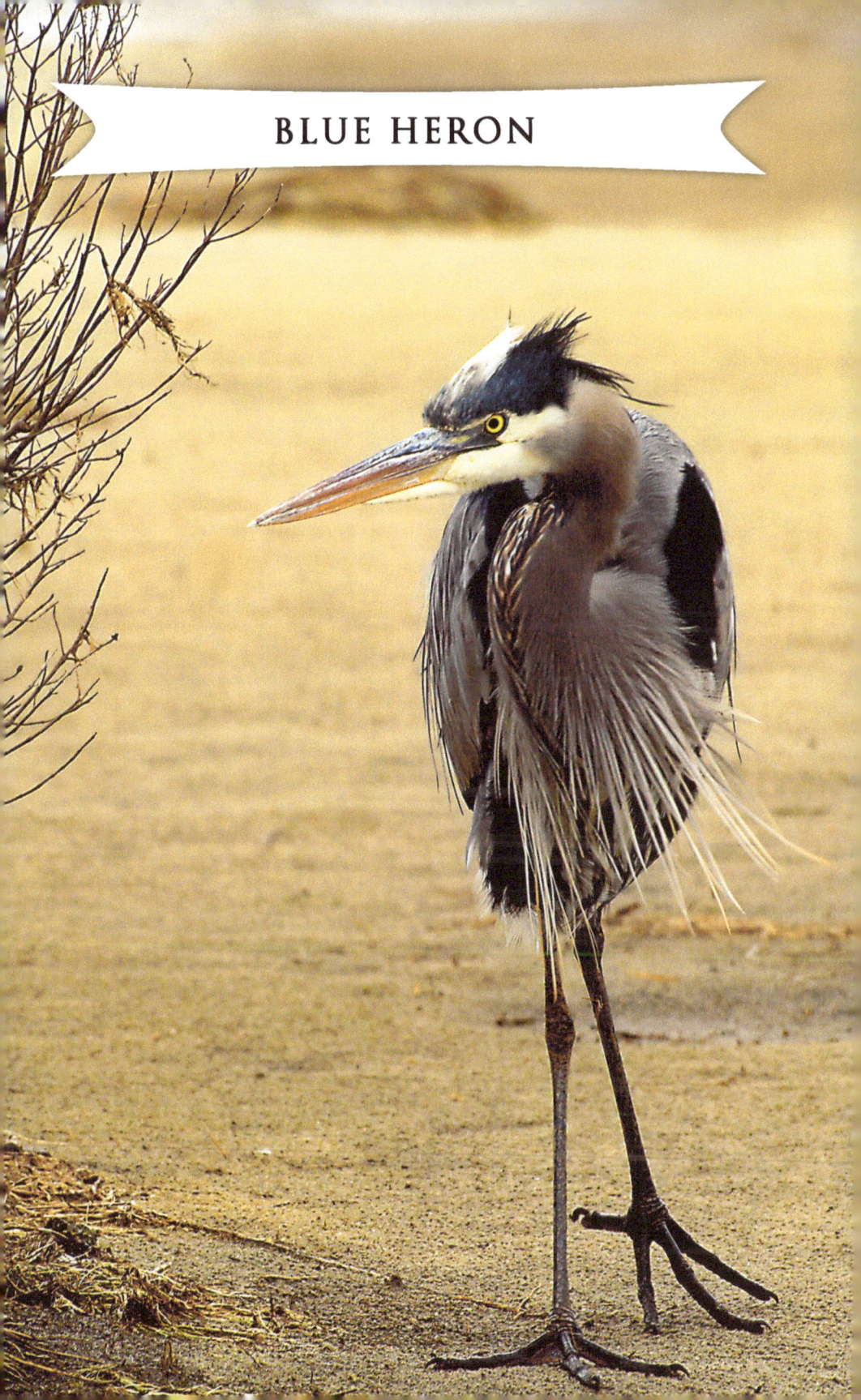

BLUE HERON

BLUE JAY

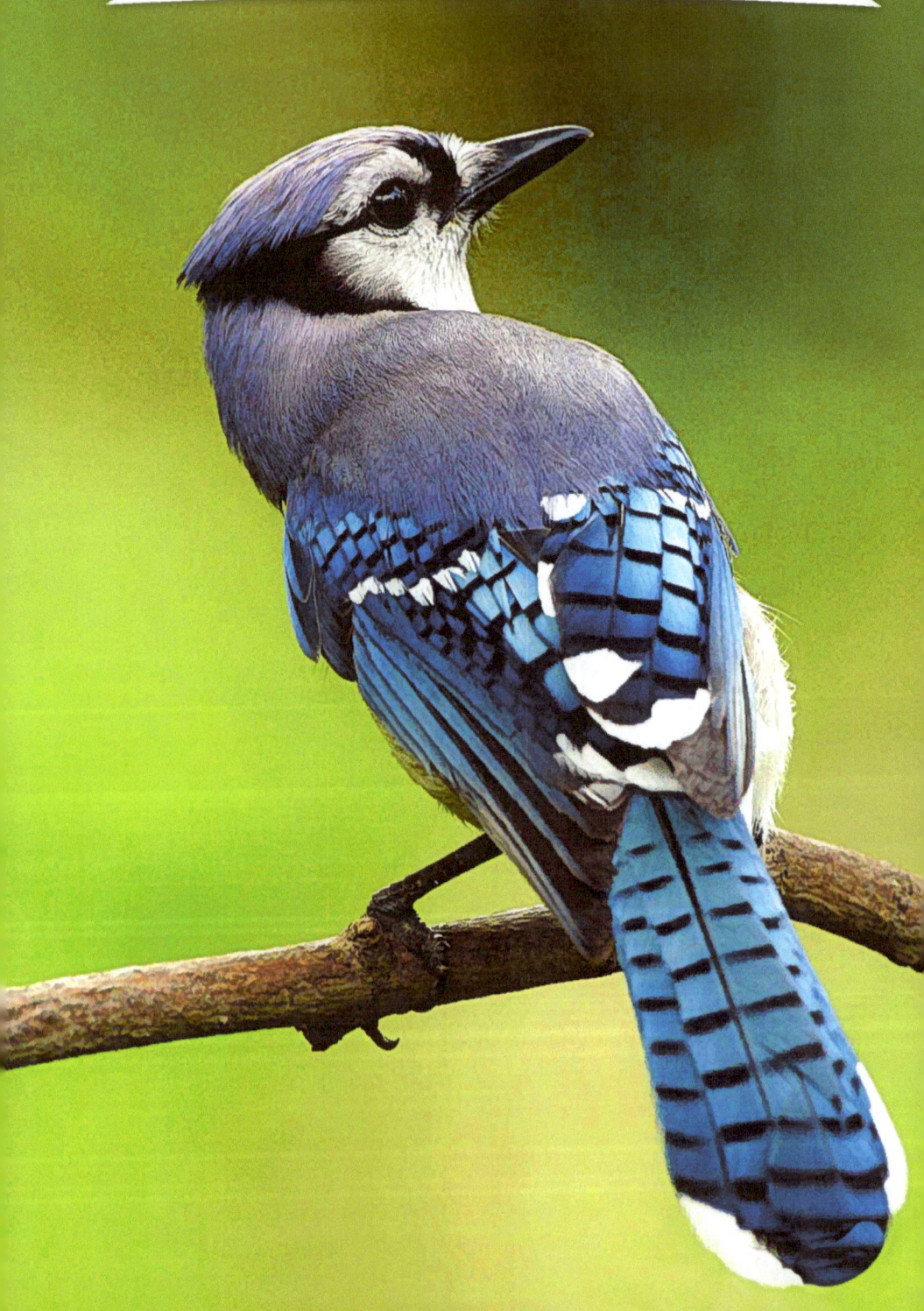

BOWERBIRD

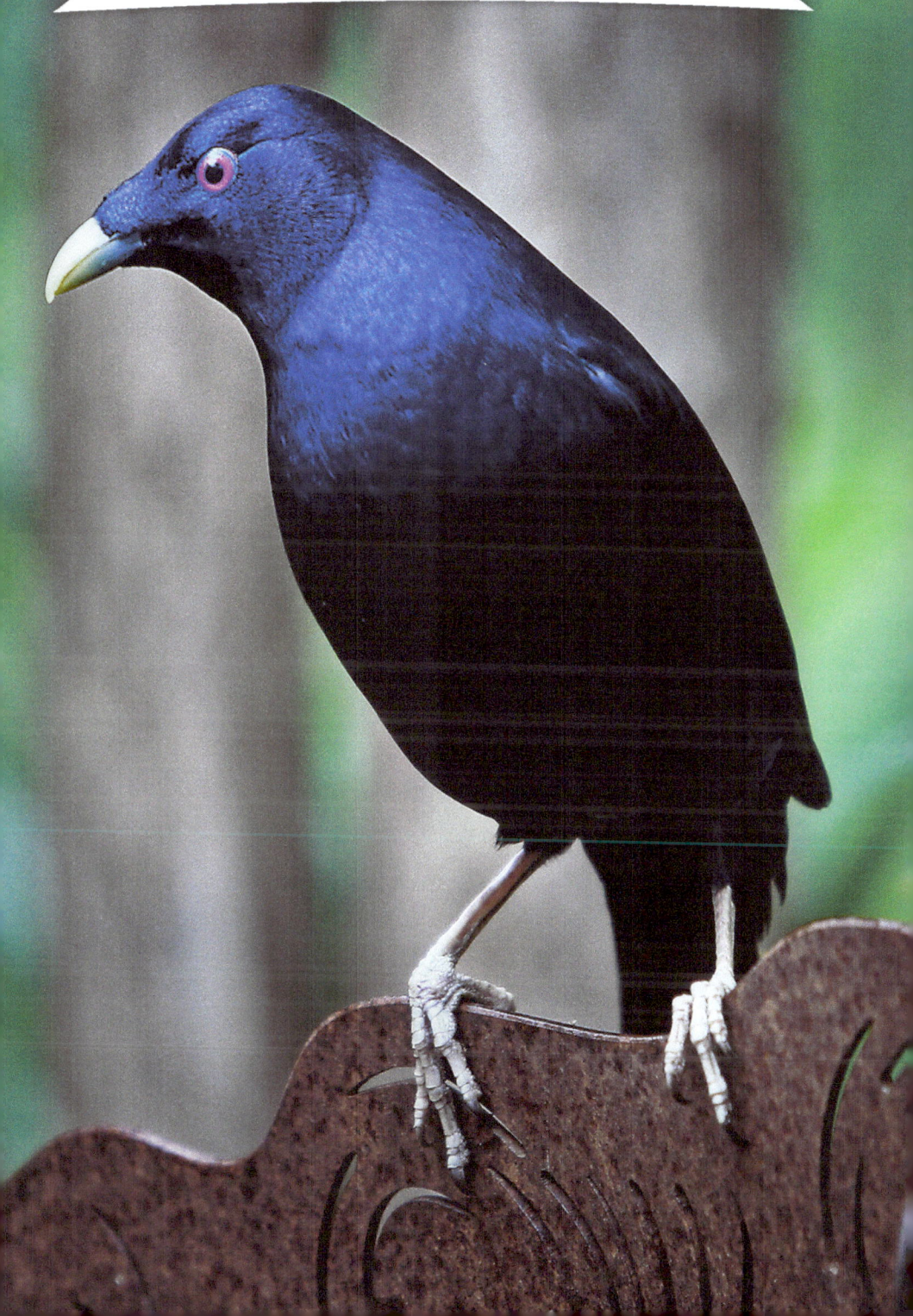

BULLFINCH

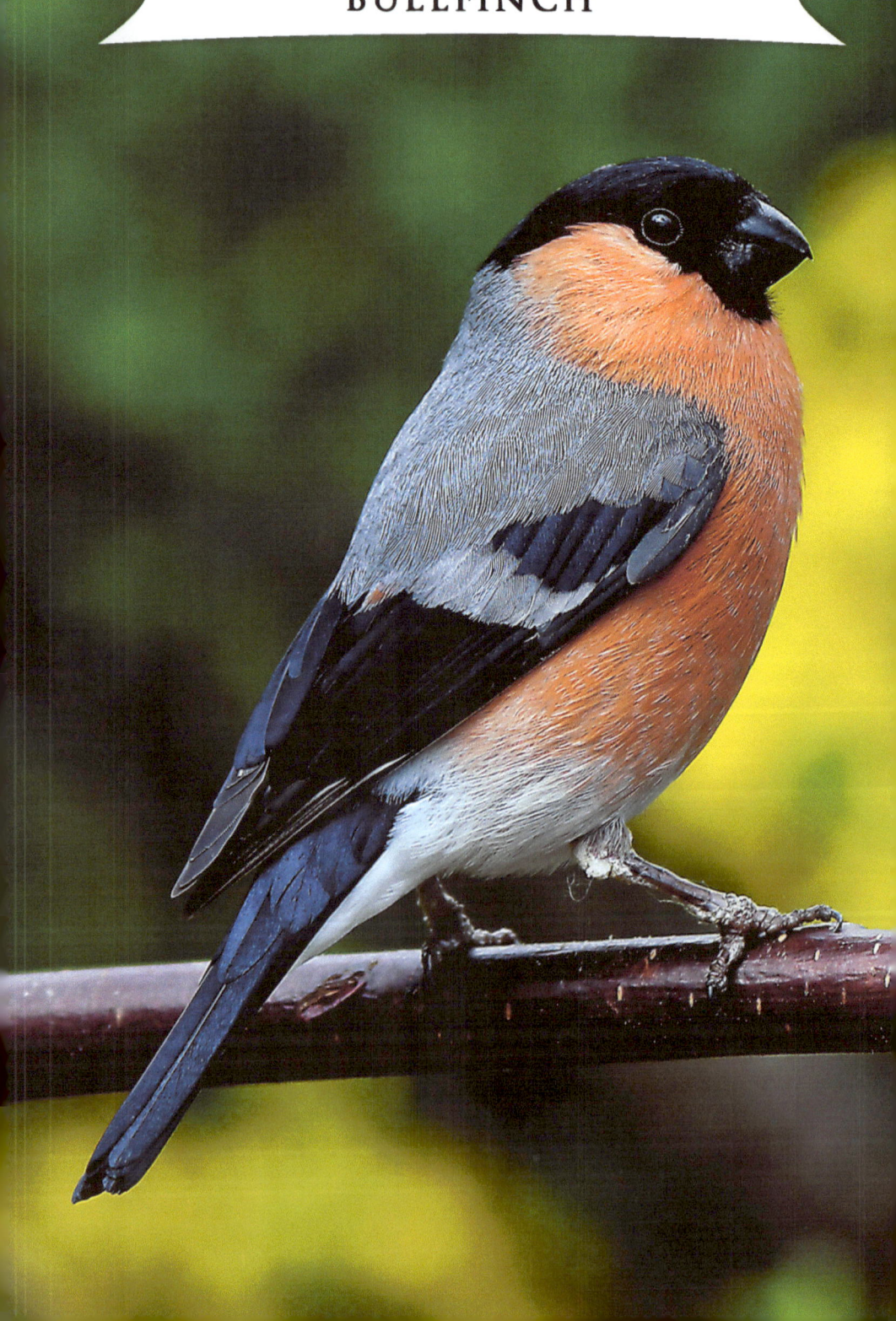

CANADA GOOSE

CARDINAL

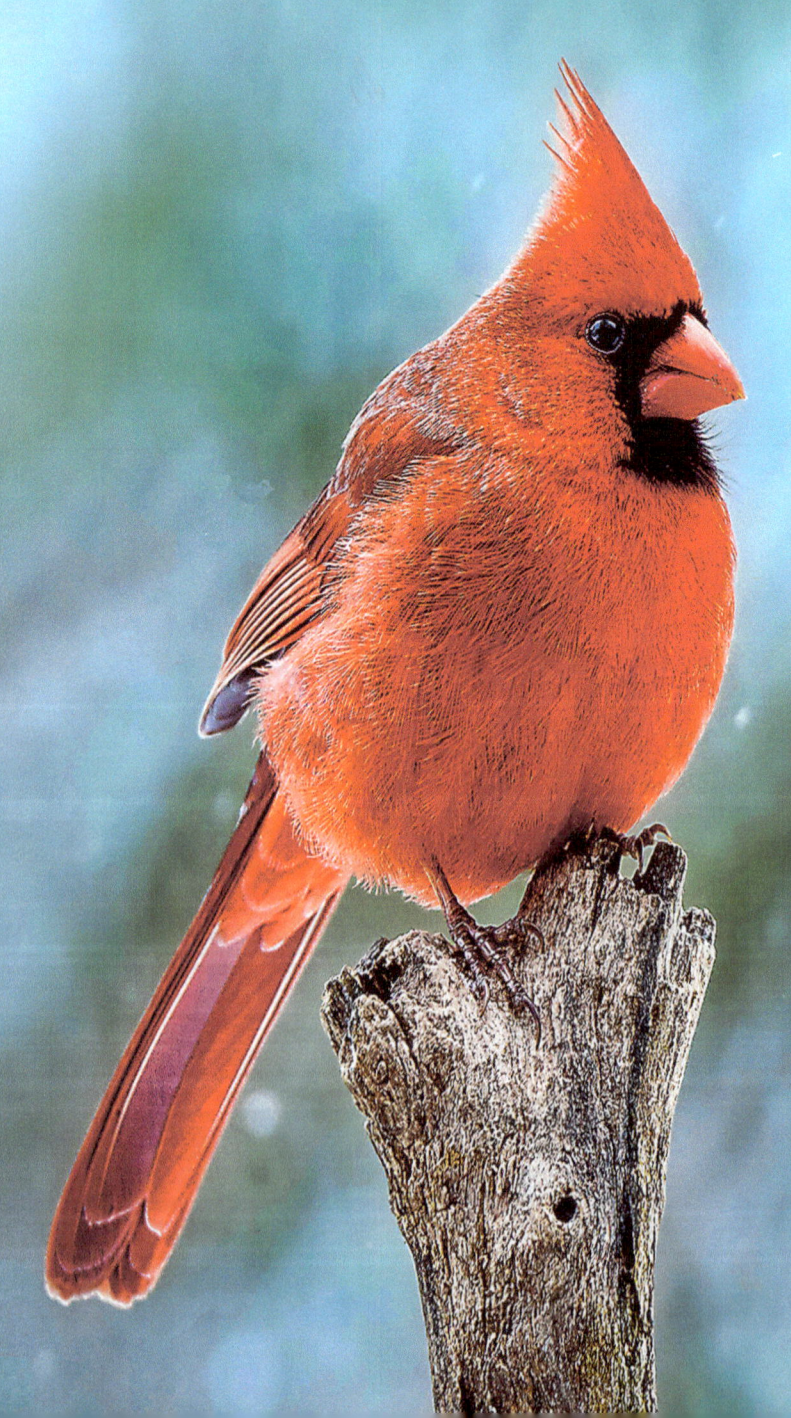

CRESTED CARA CARA

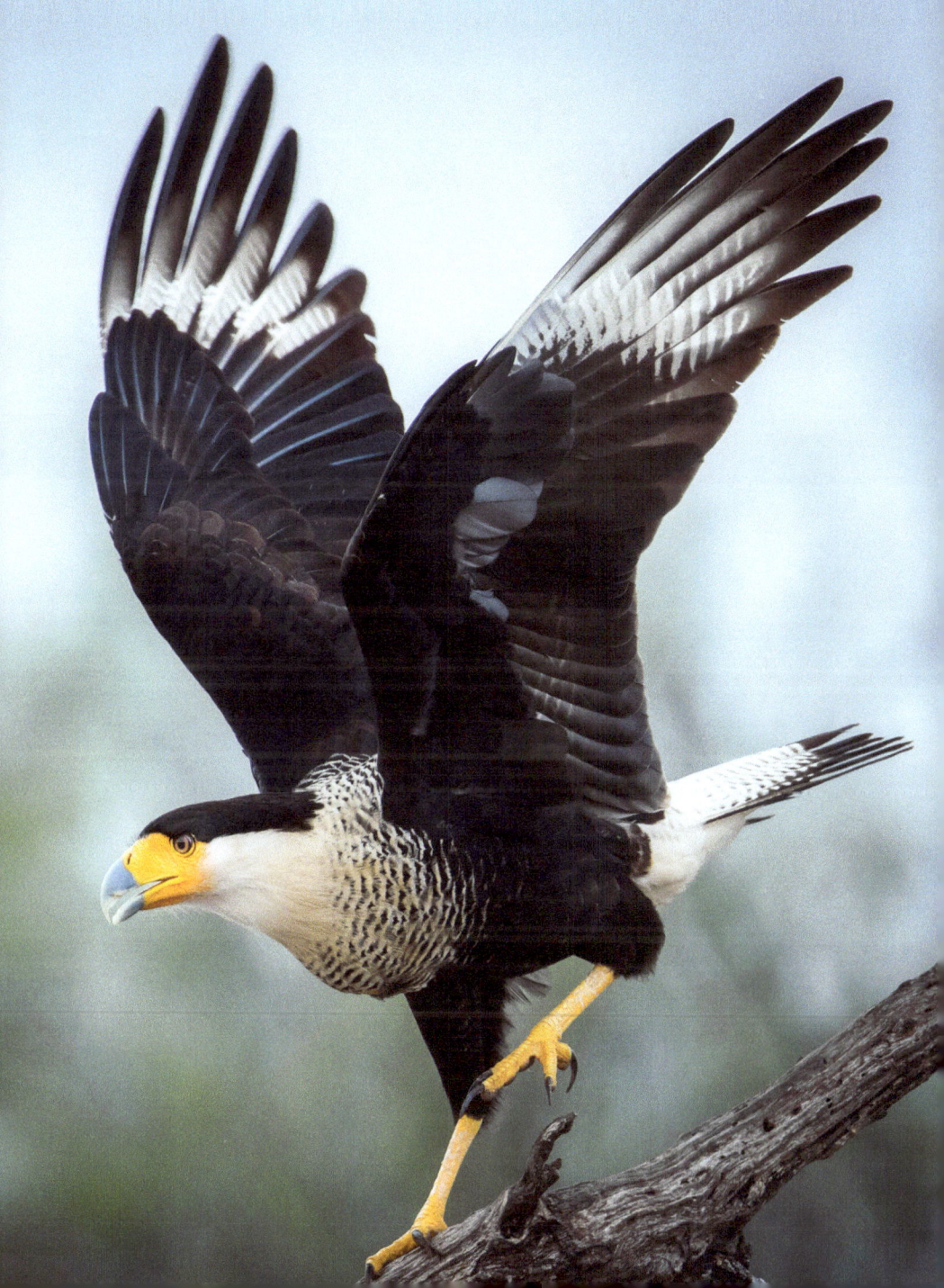

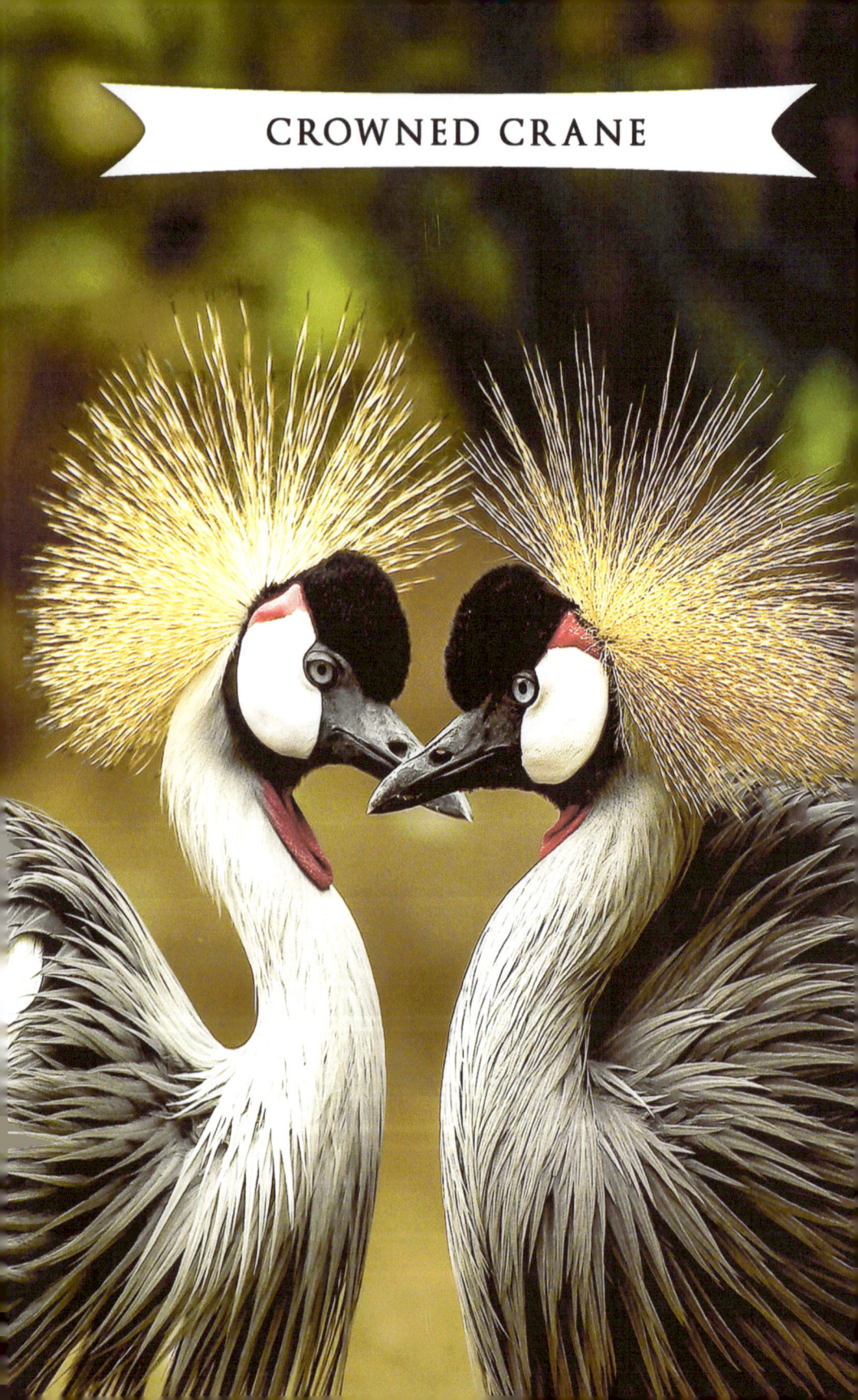

CROWNED CRANE

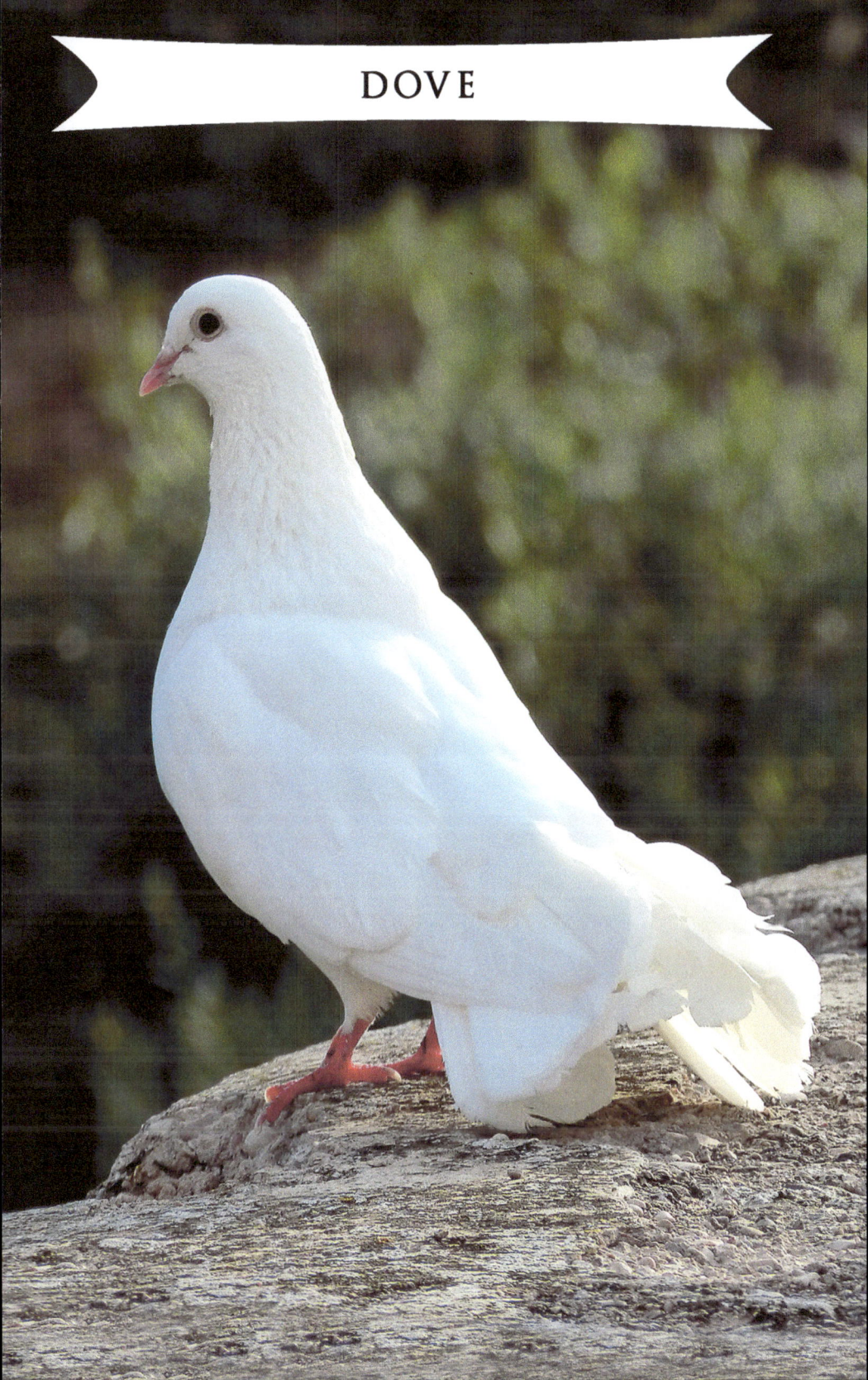

DOVE

EAGLE

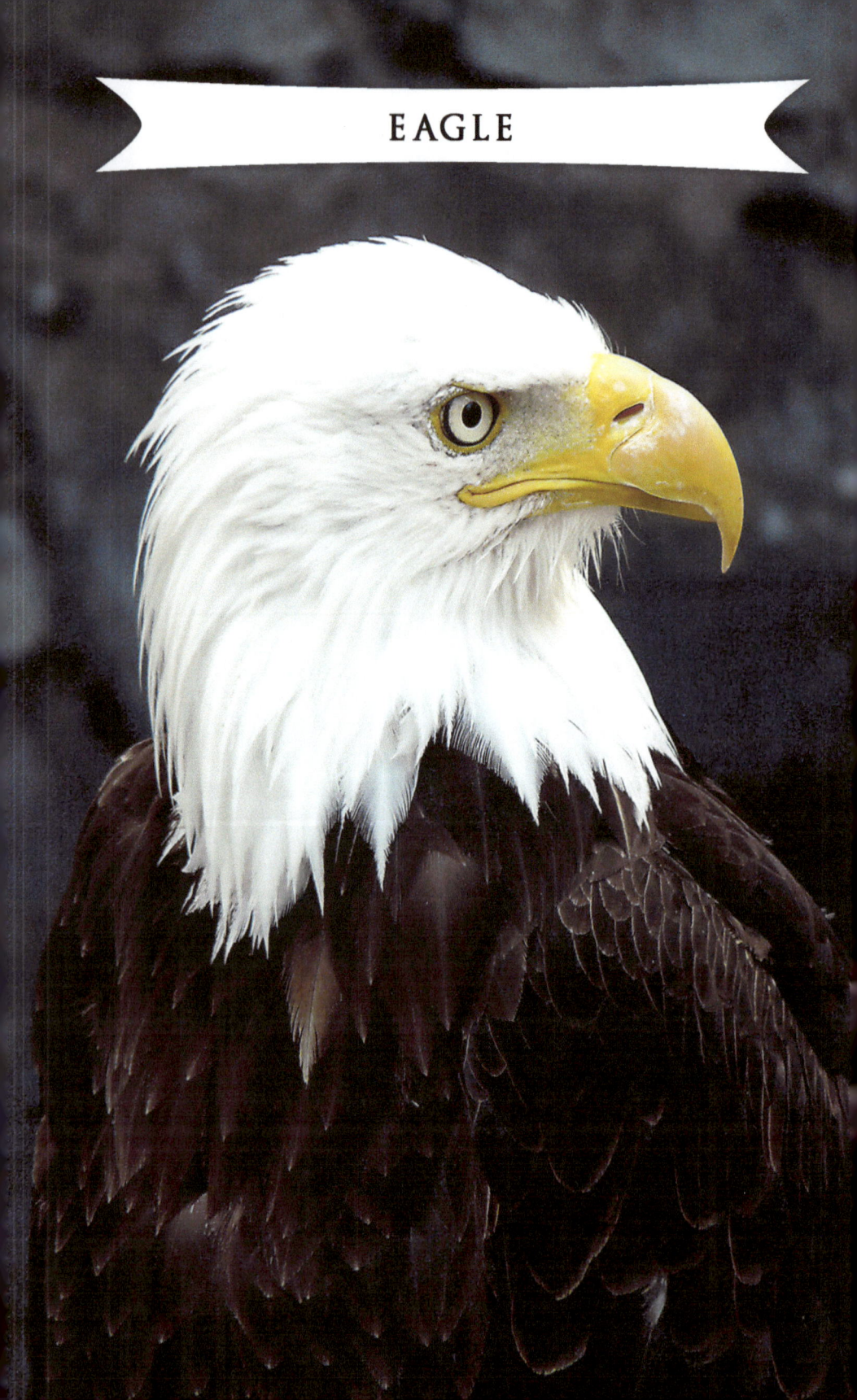

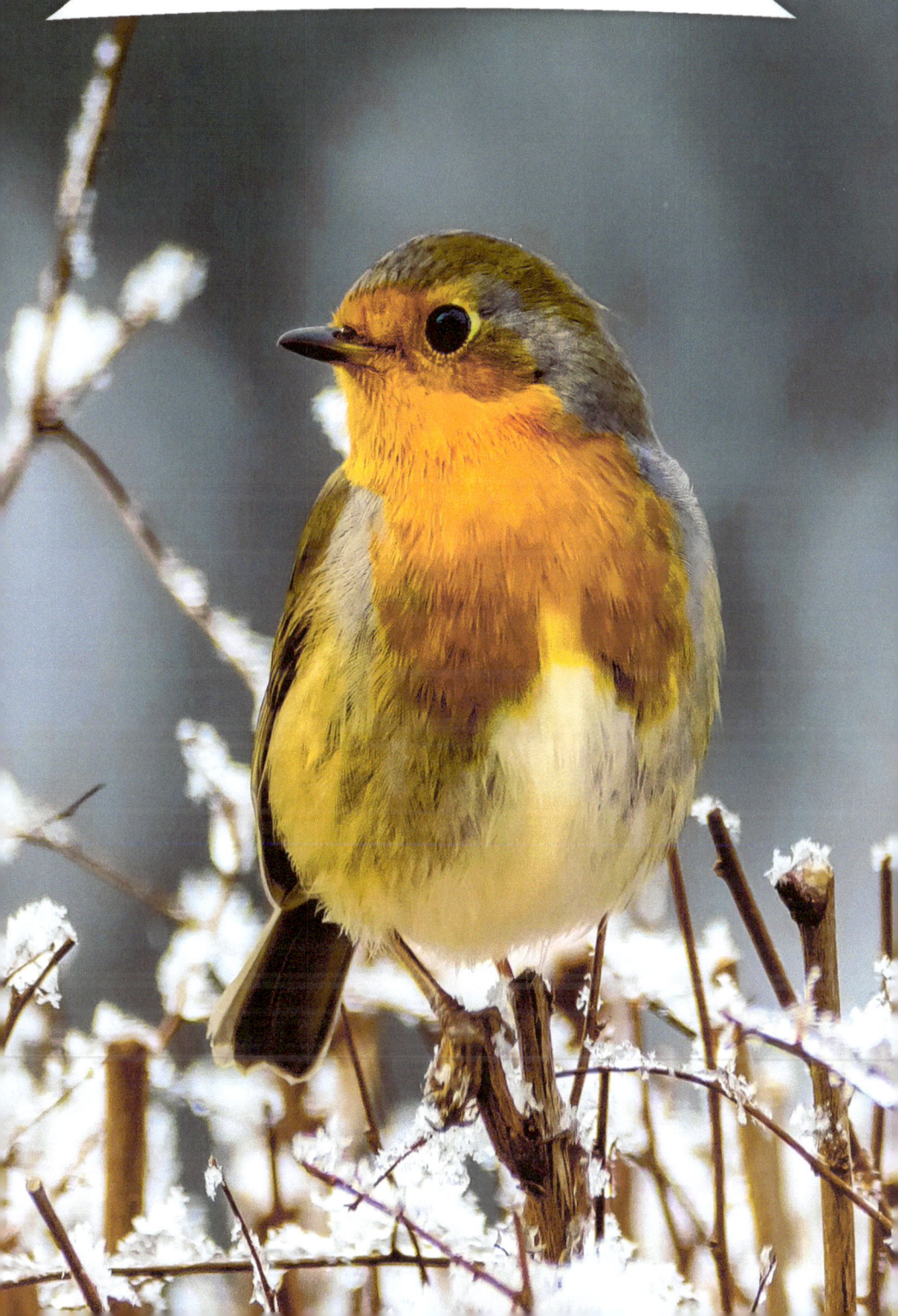

EUROPEAN ROBIN

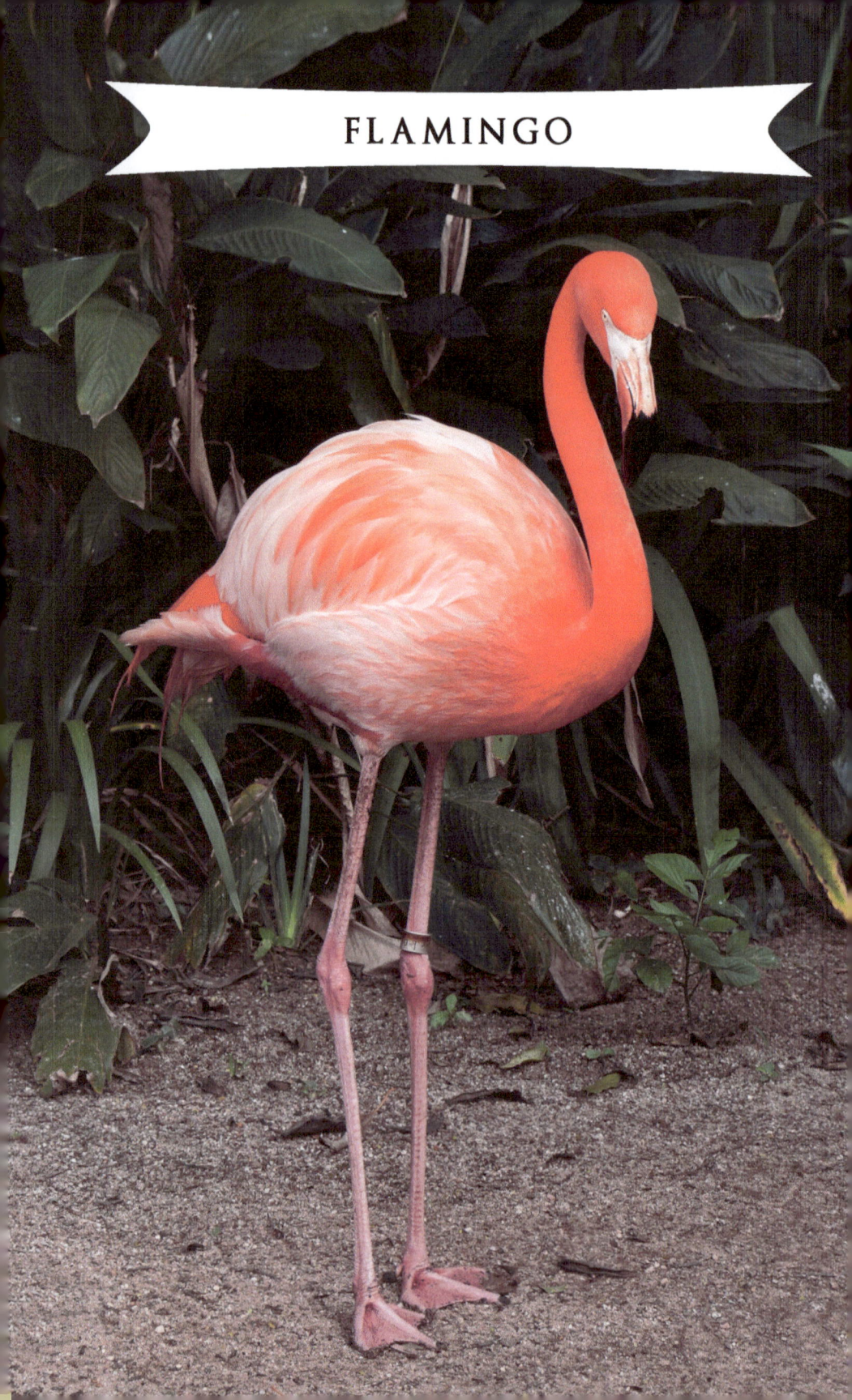

FLAMINGO

GOLDFINCH

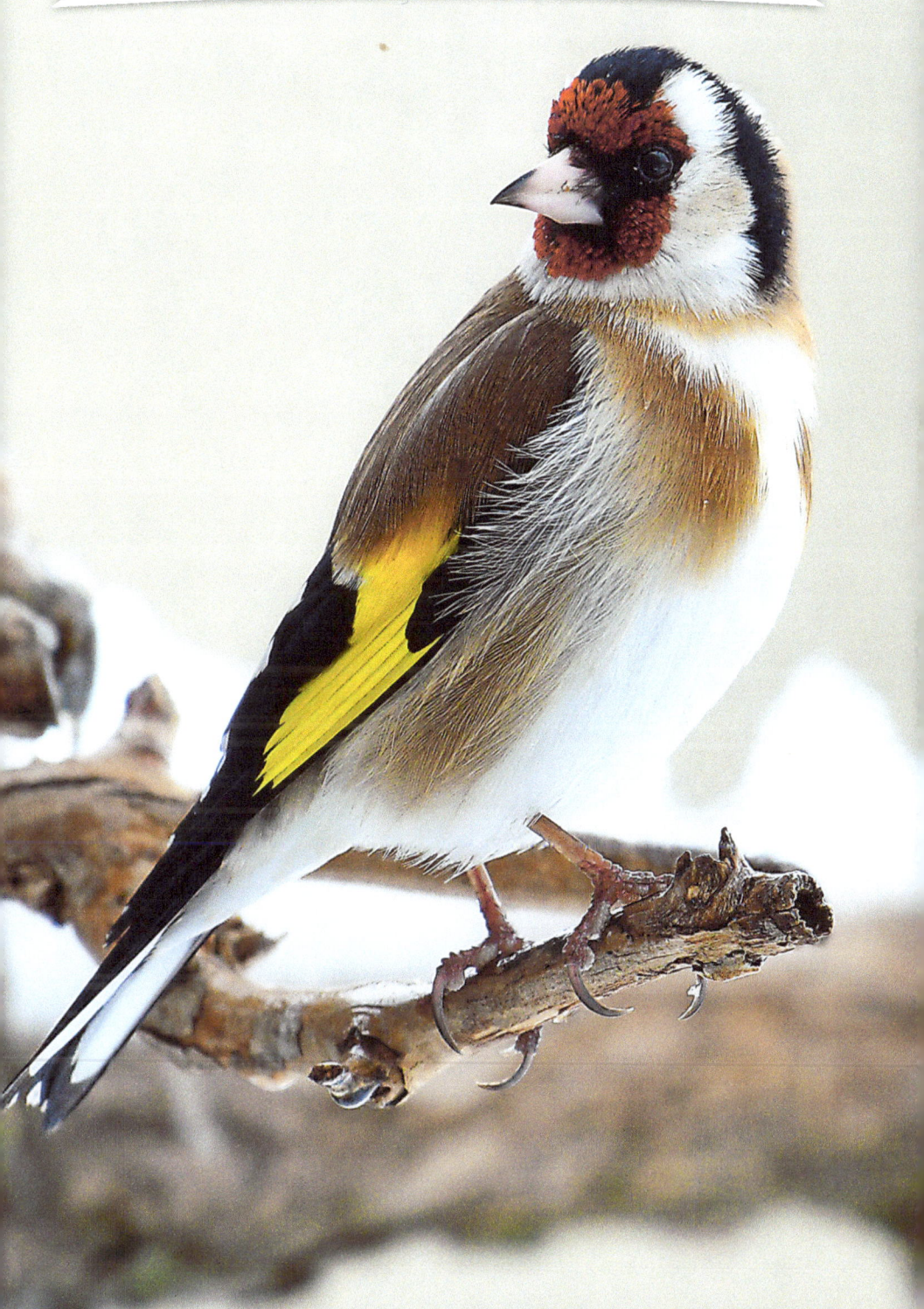

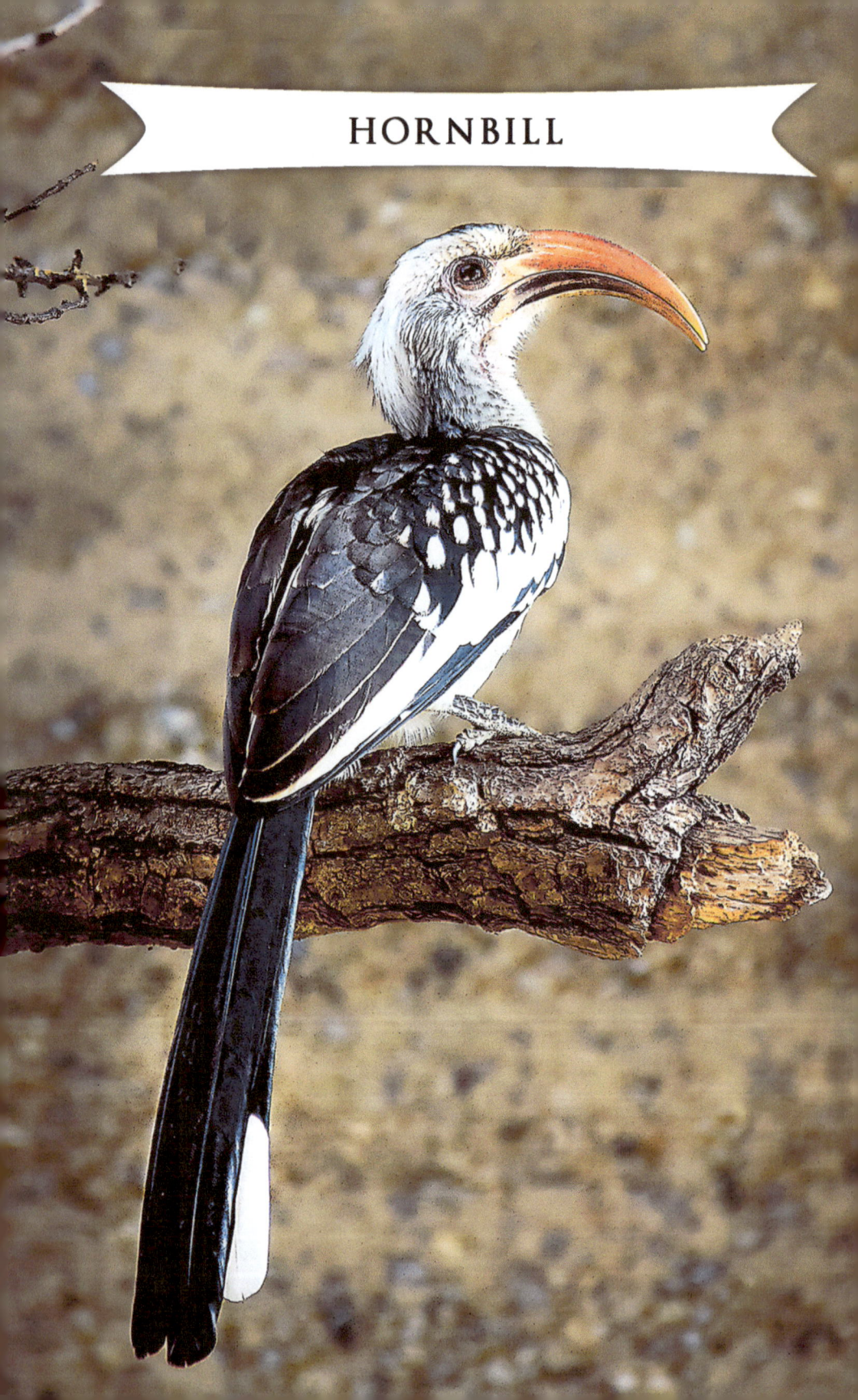

HORNBILL

HUMMINGBIRD

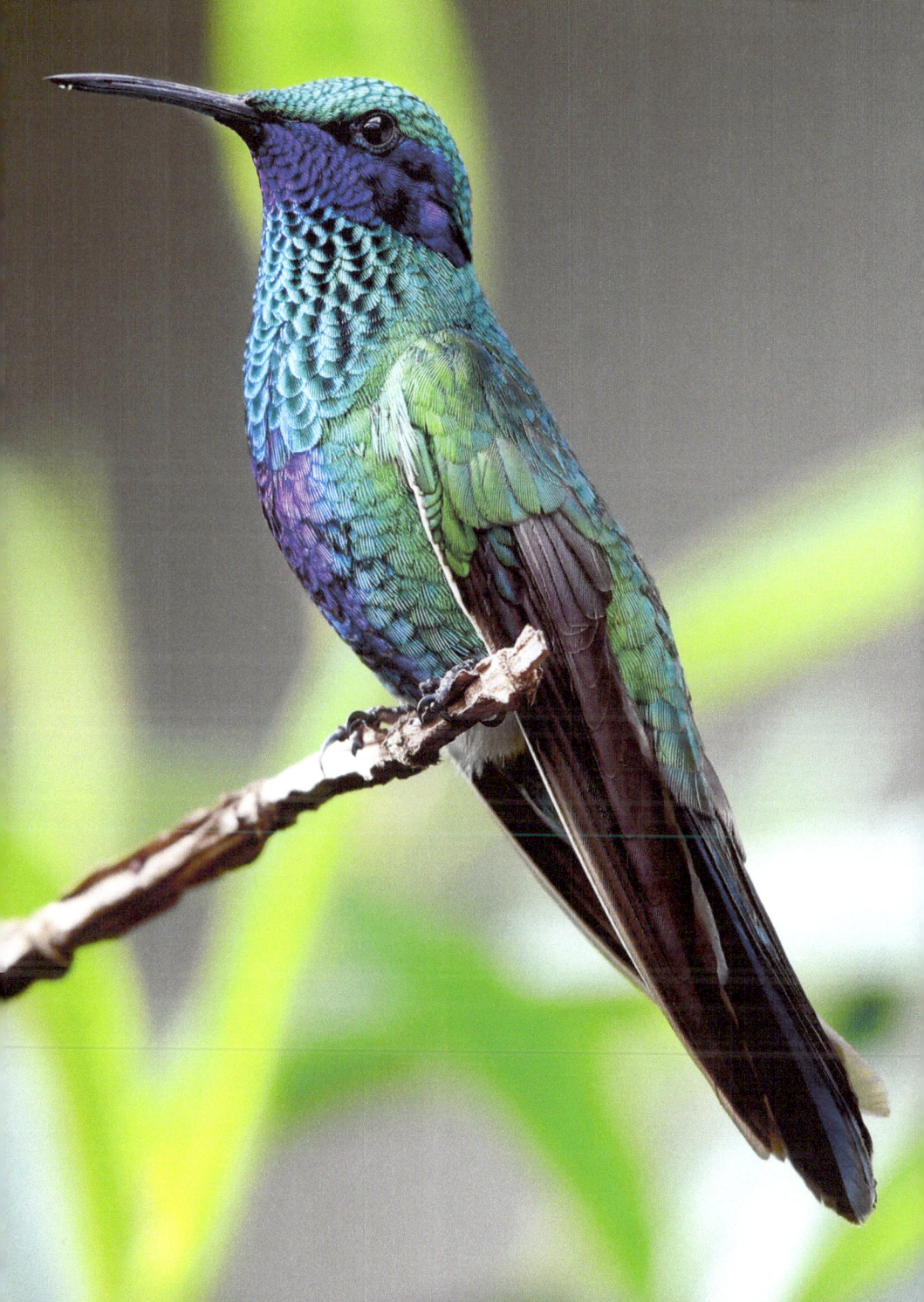

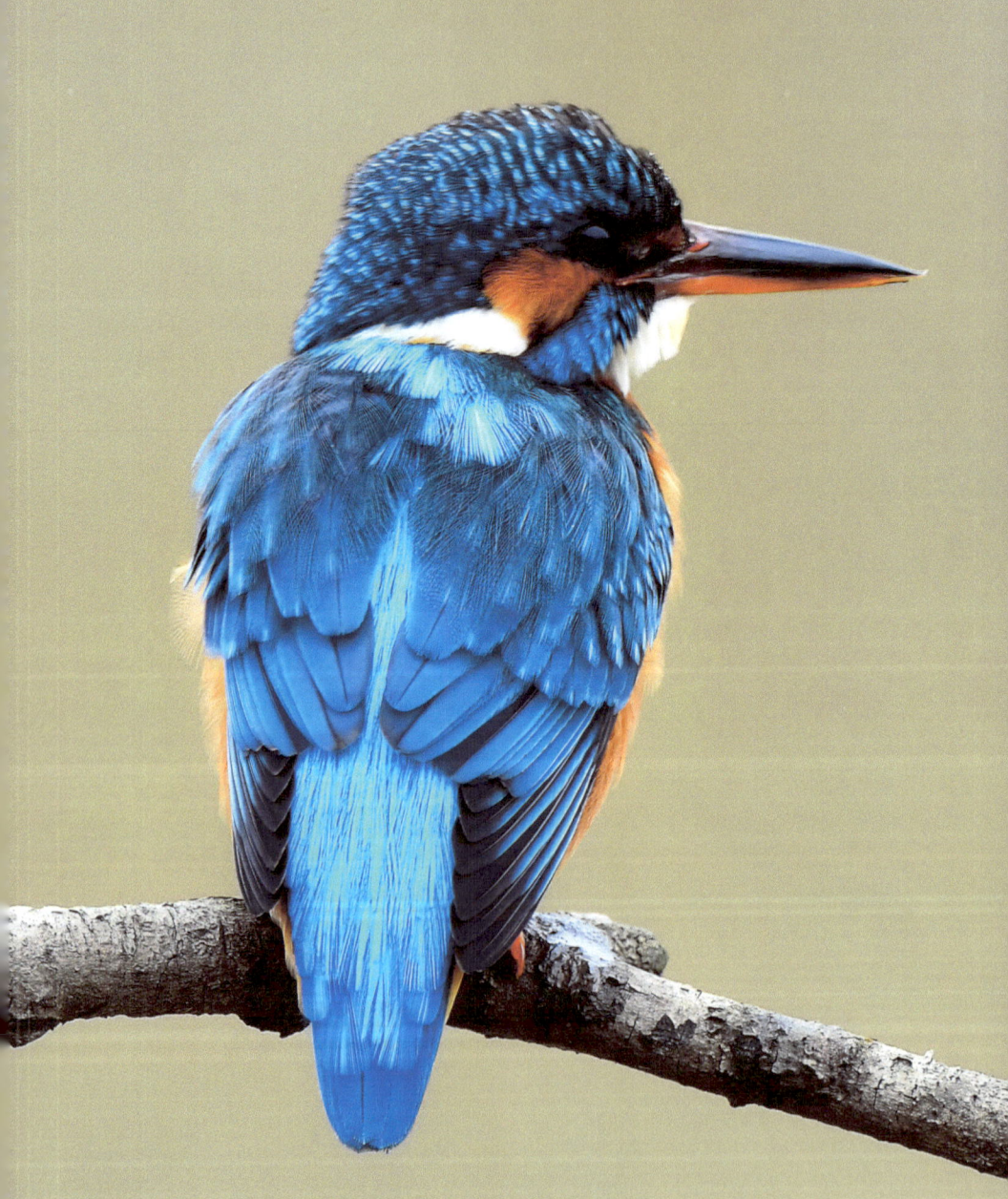

LORIKEET

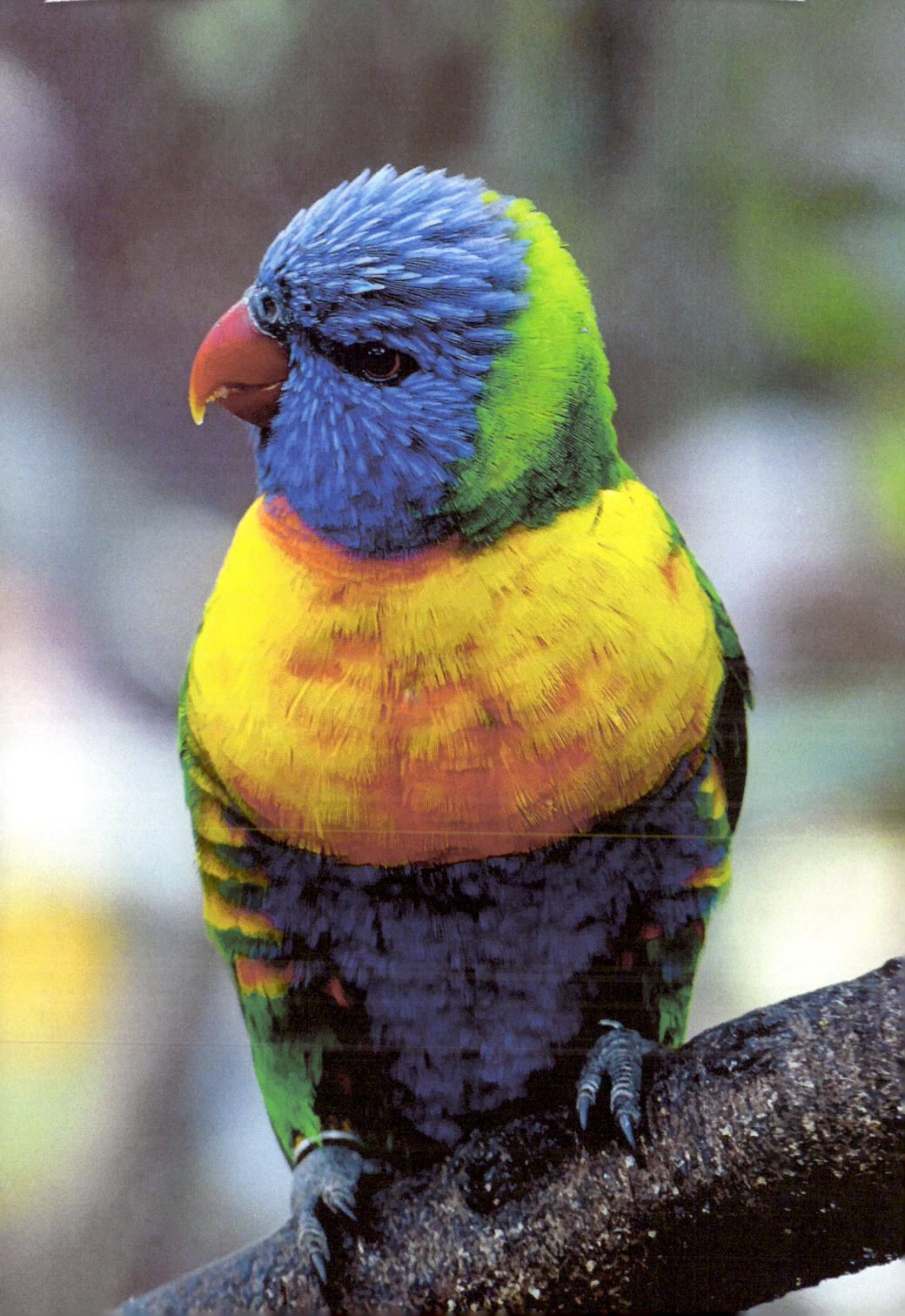

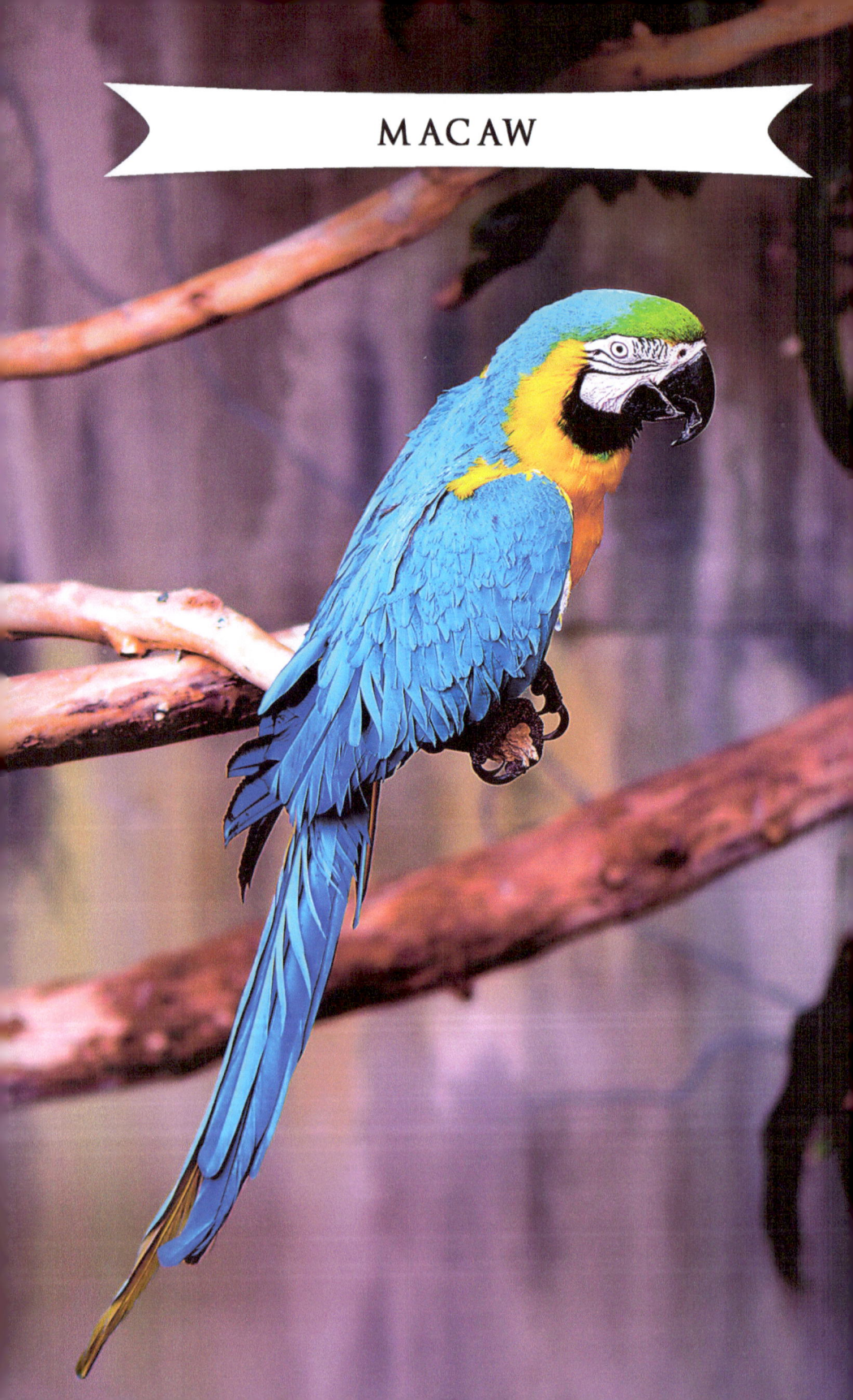

MACAW

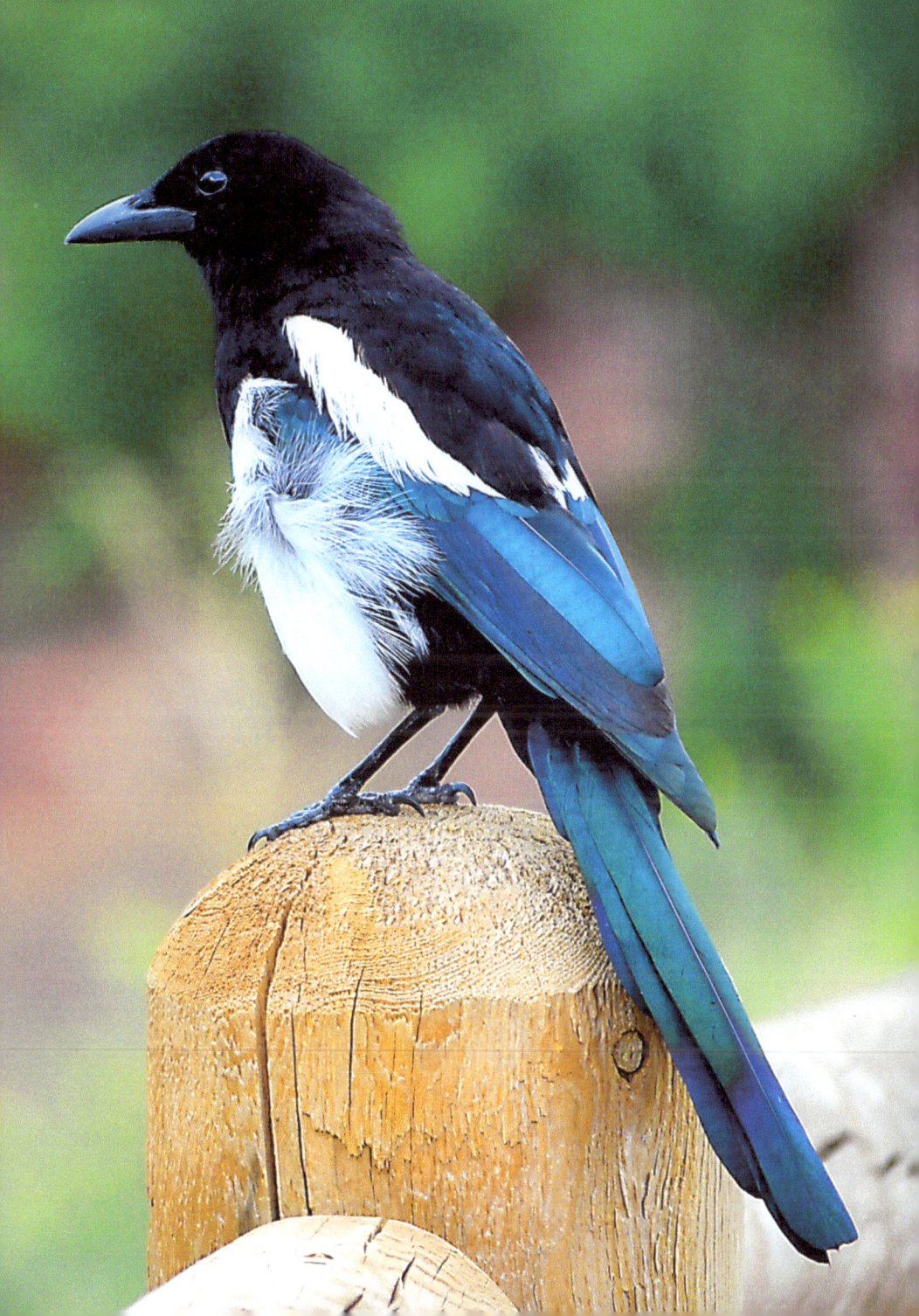

MAGPIE

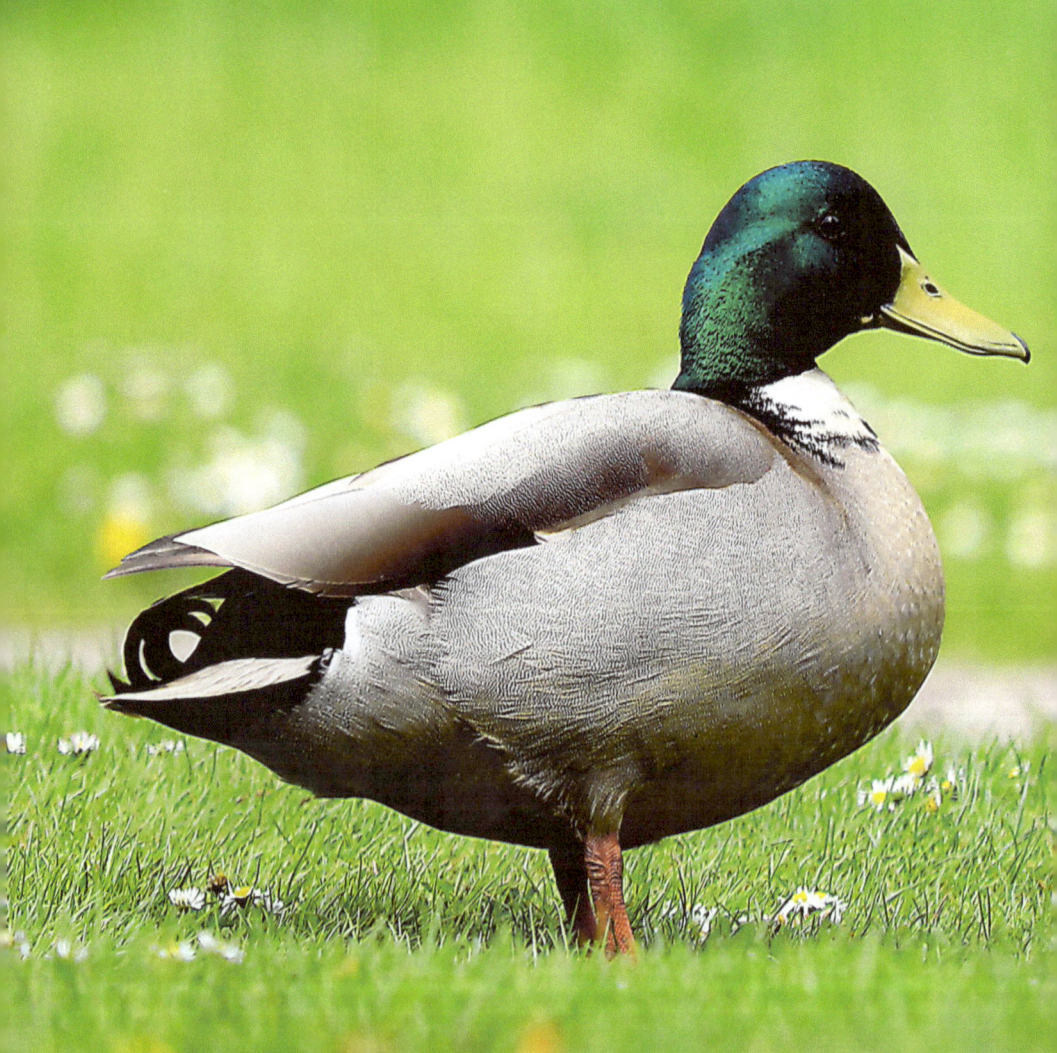

MALLARD DUCK

MANDARIN DUCK

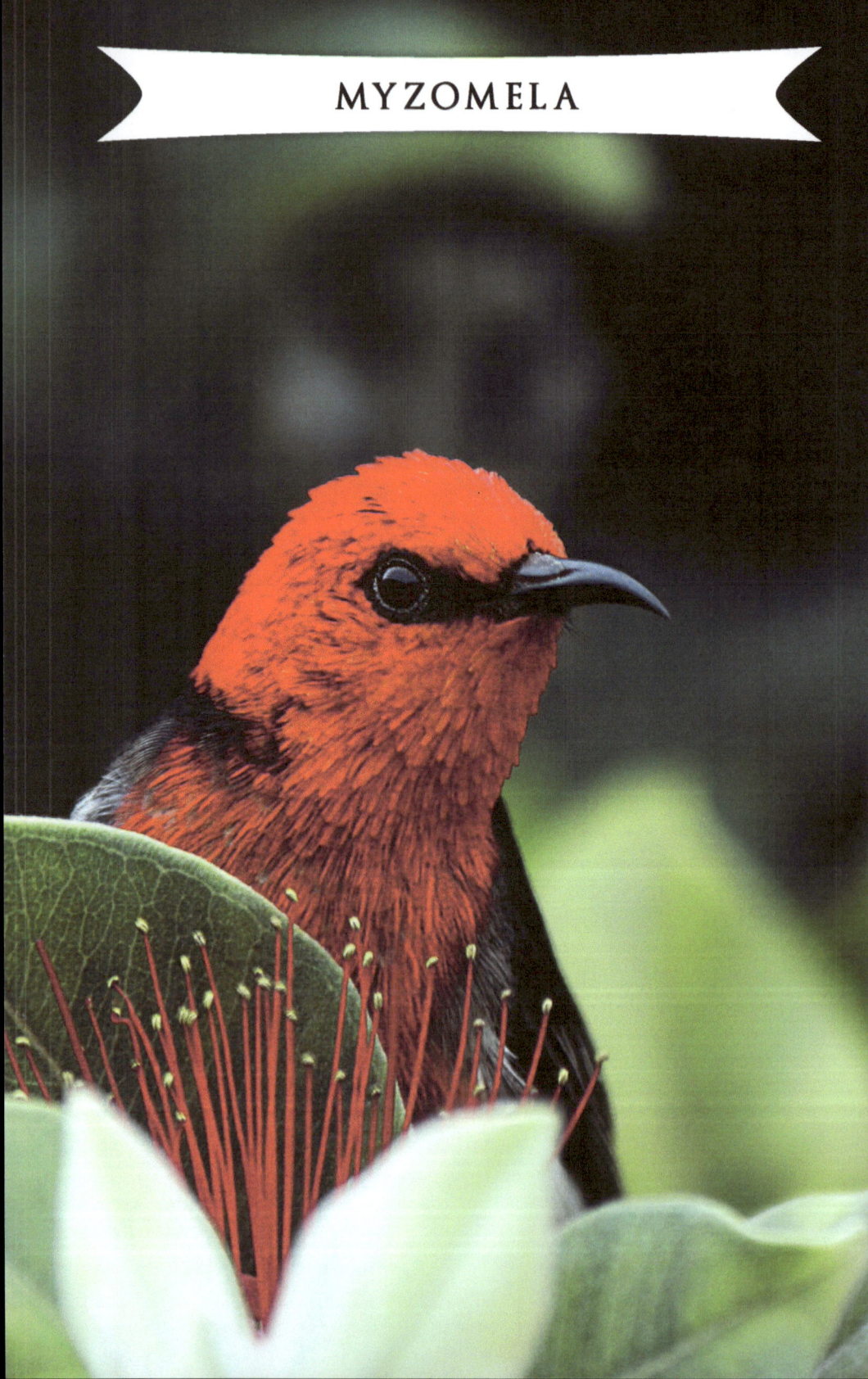

OSPREY

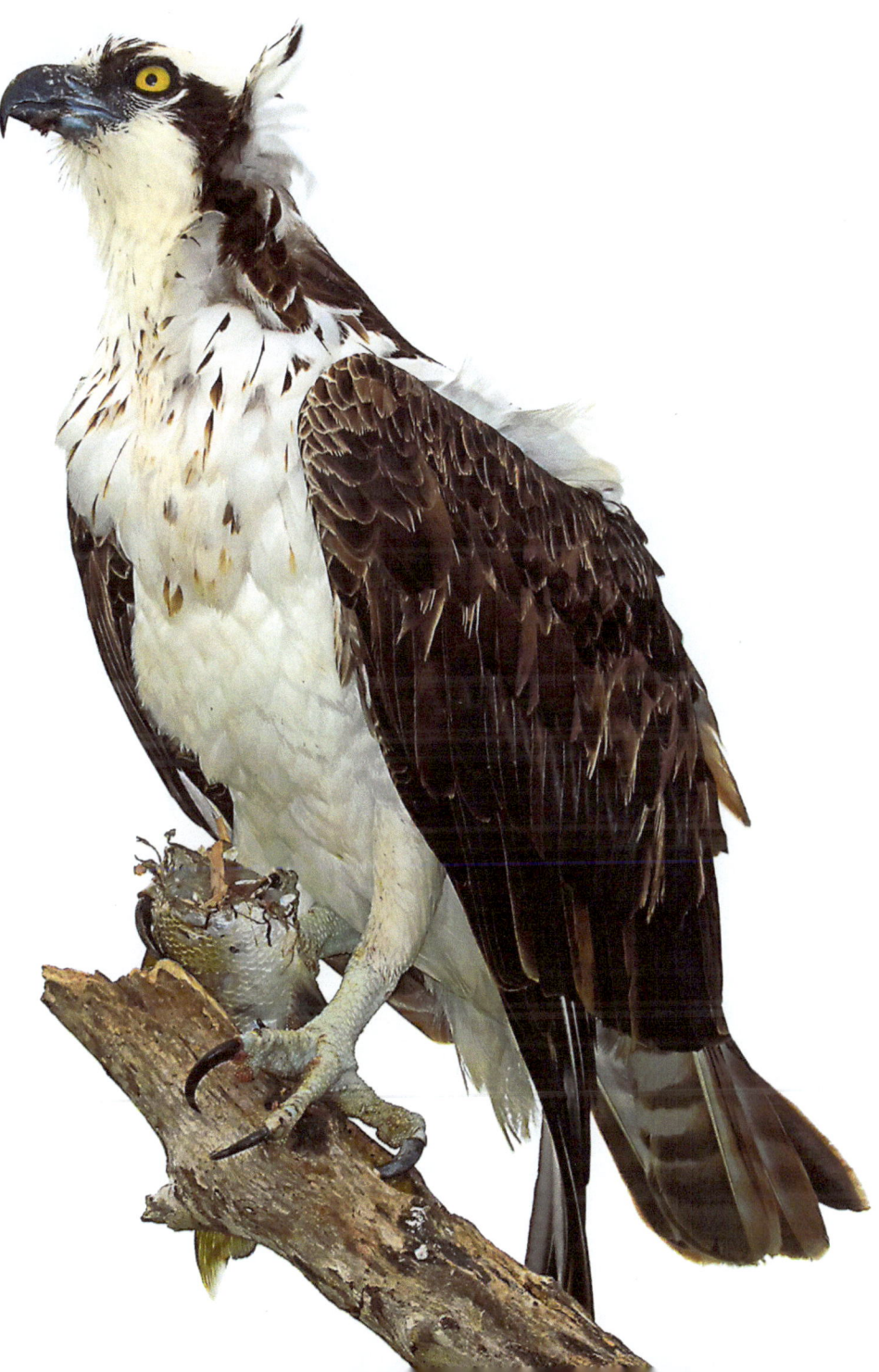

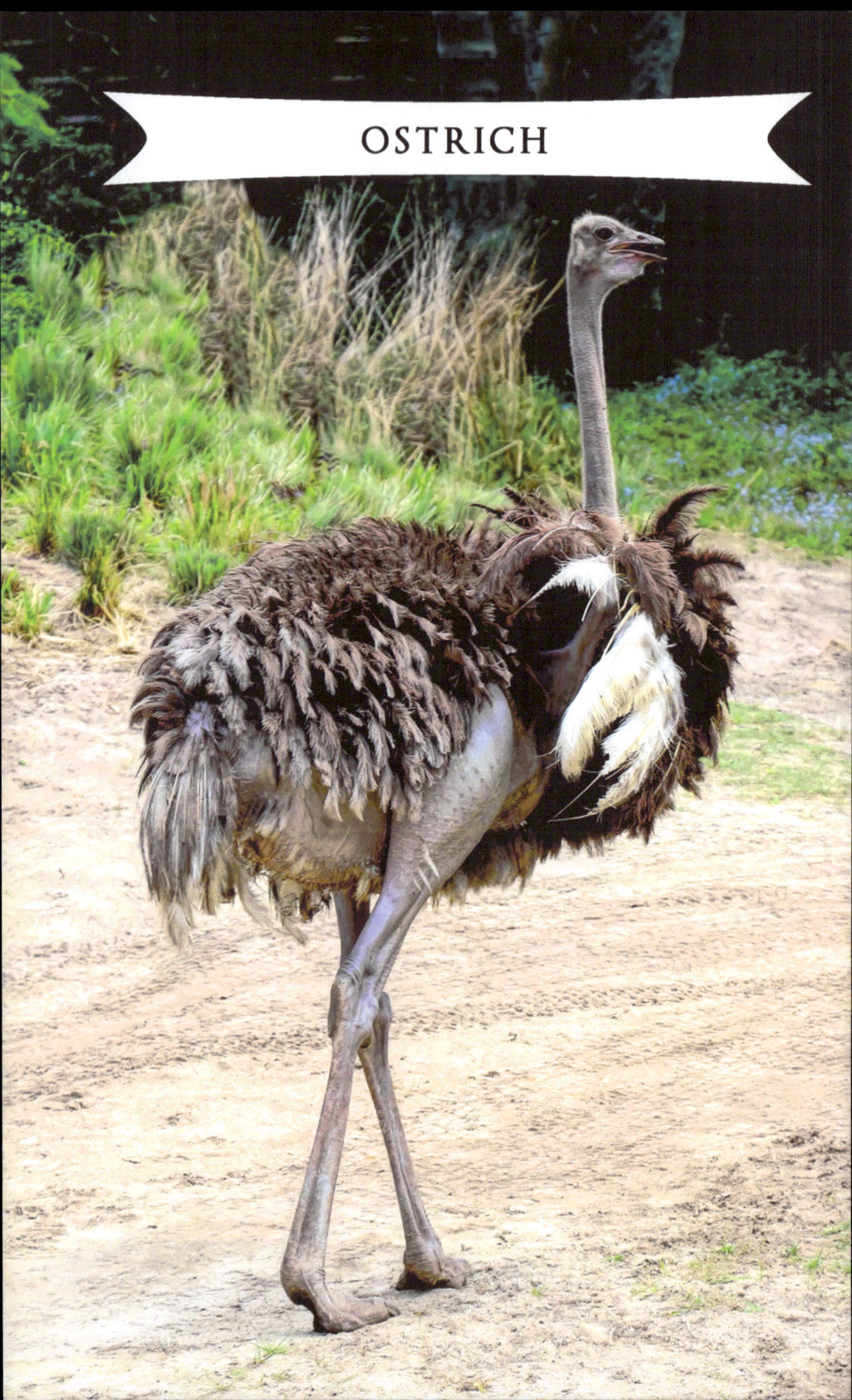

OSTRICH

PARAKEET

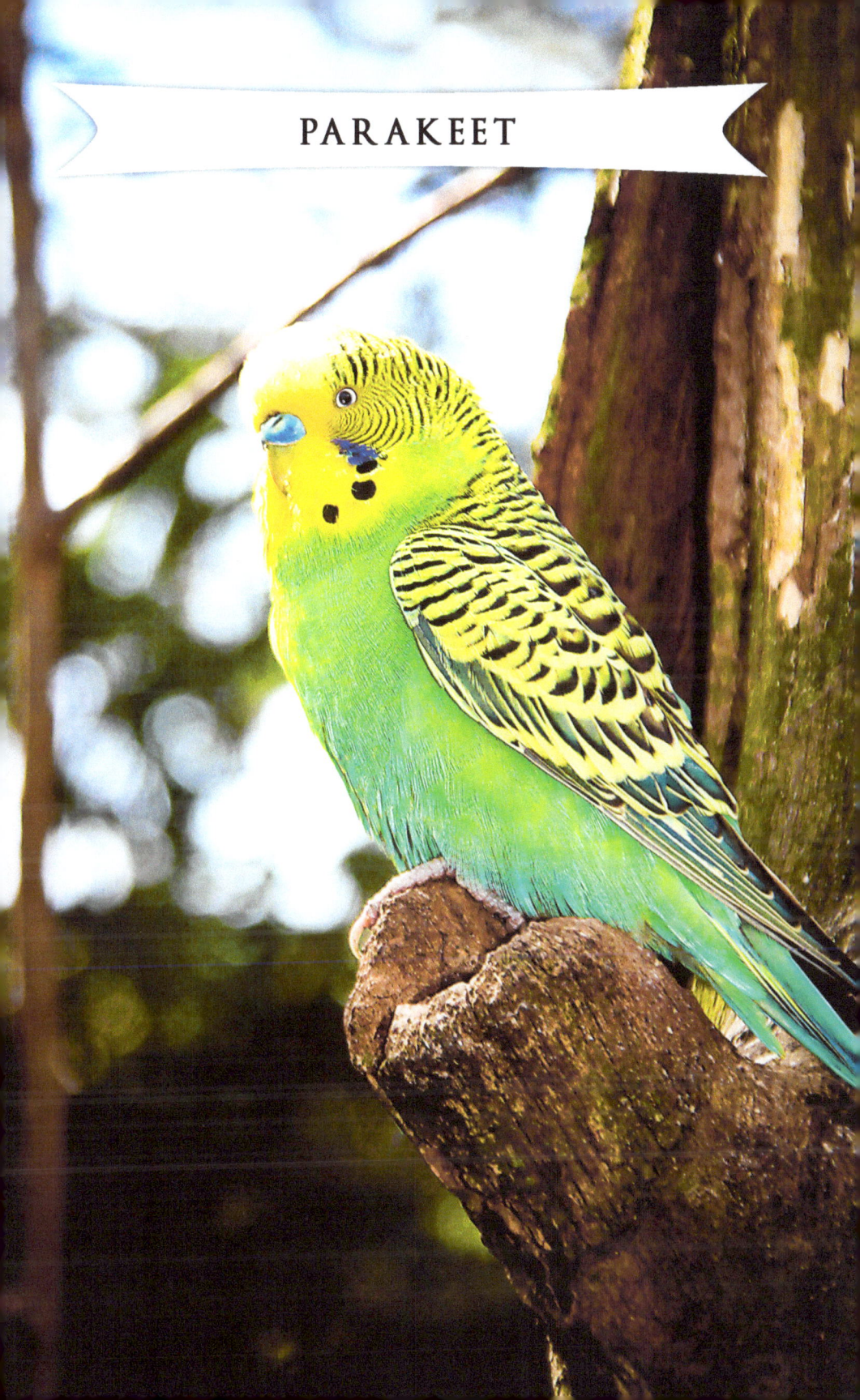

PARROT

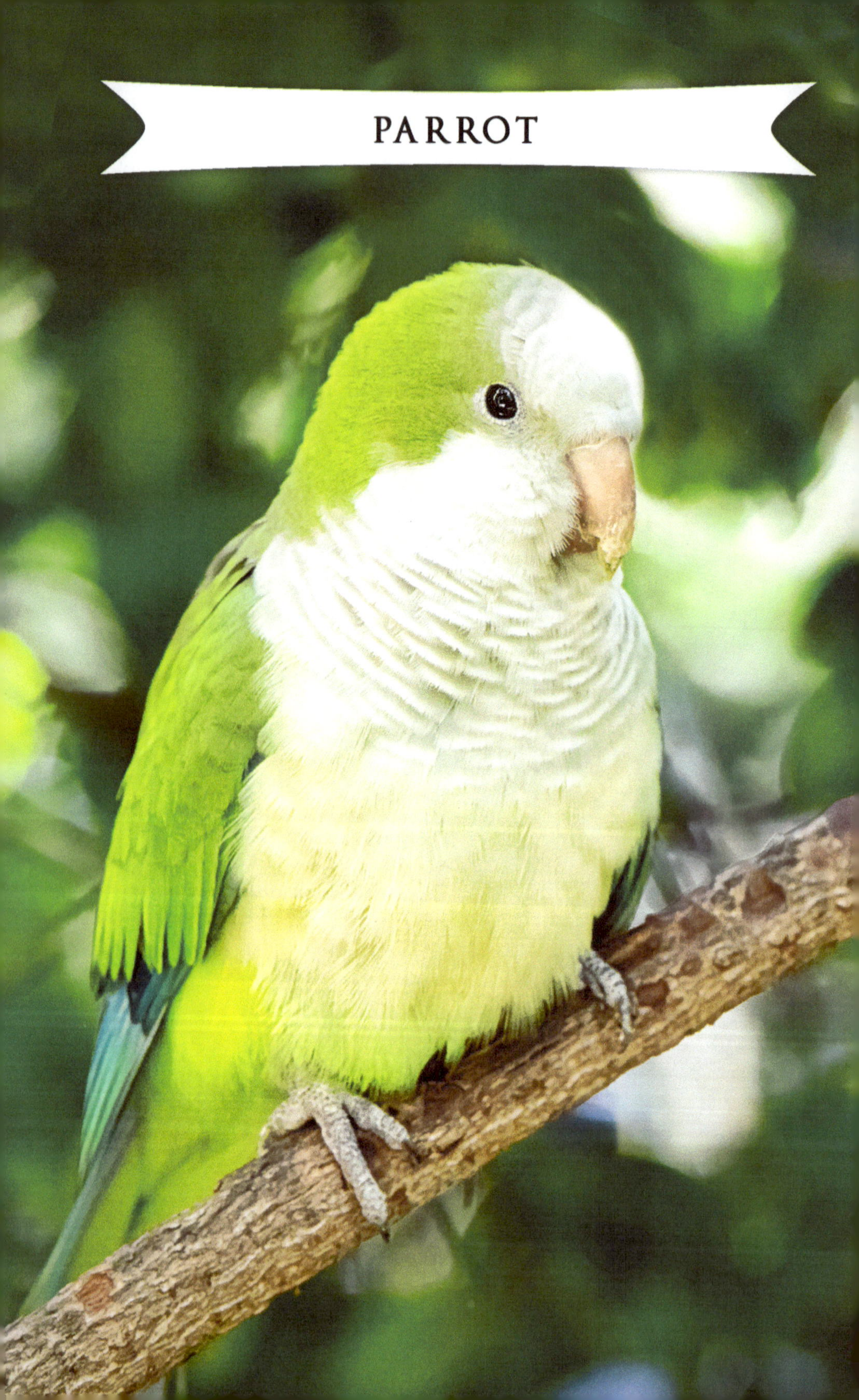

PEACOCK

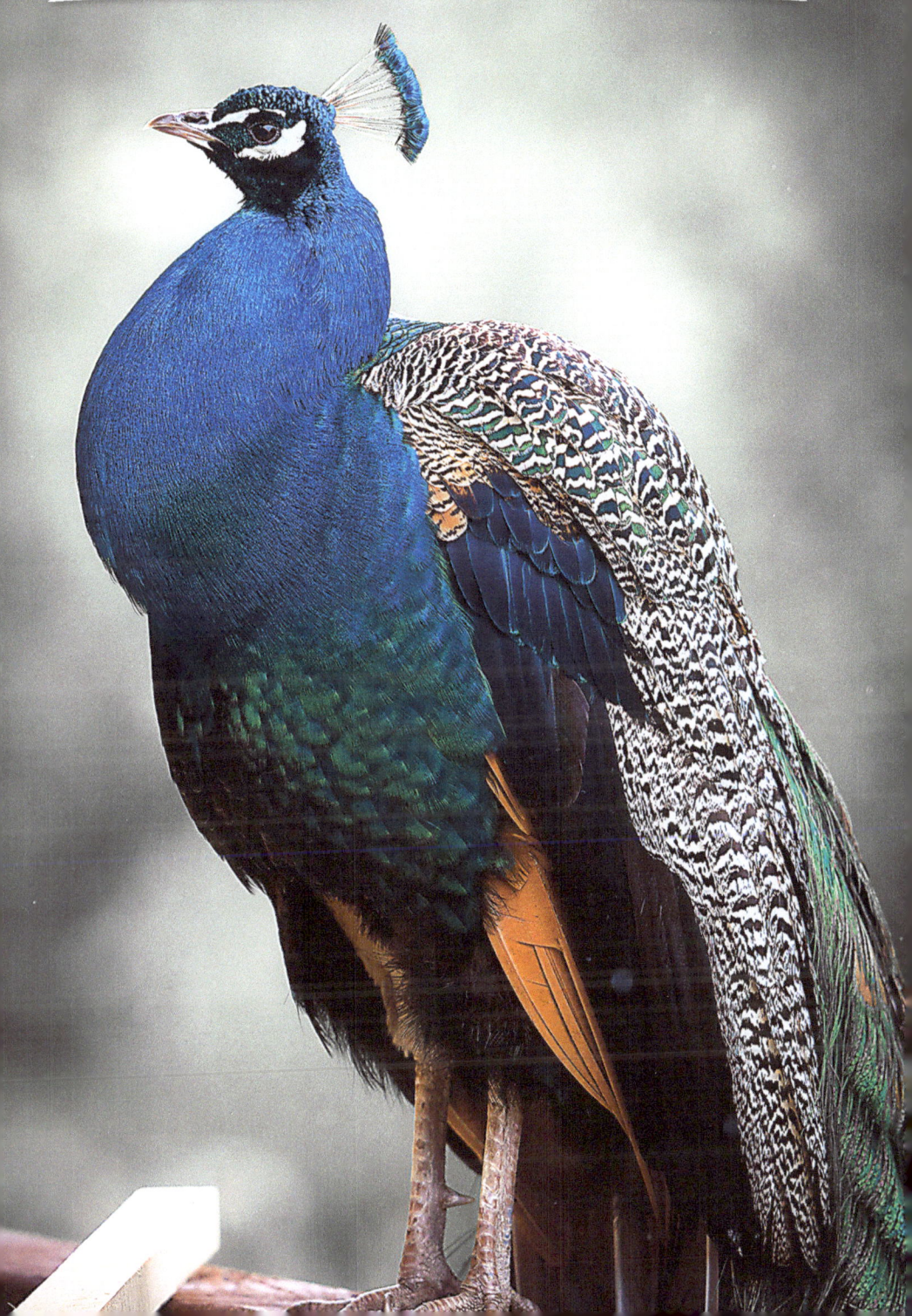

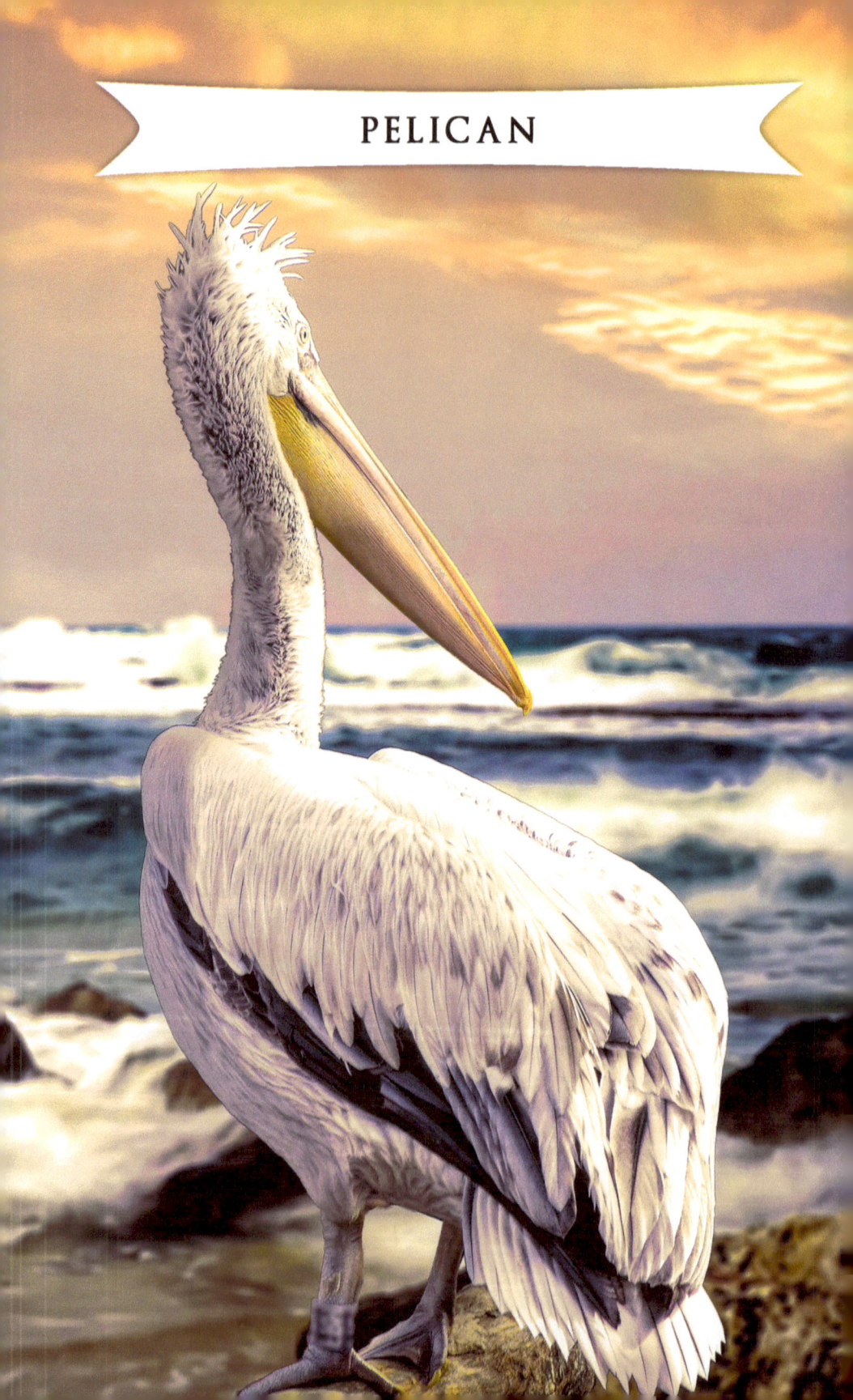

PELICAN

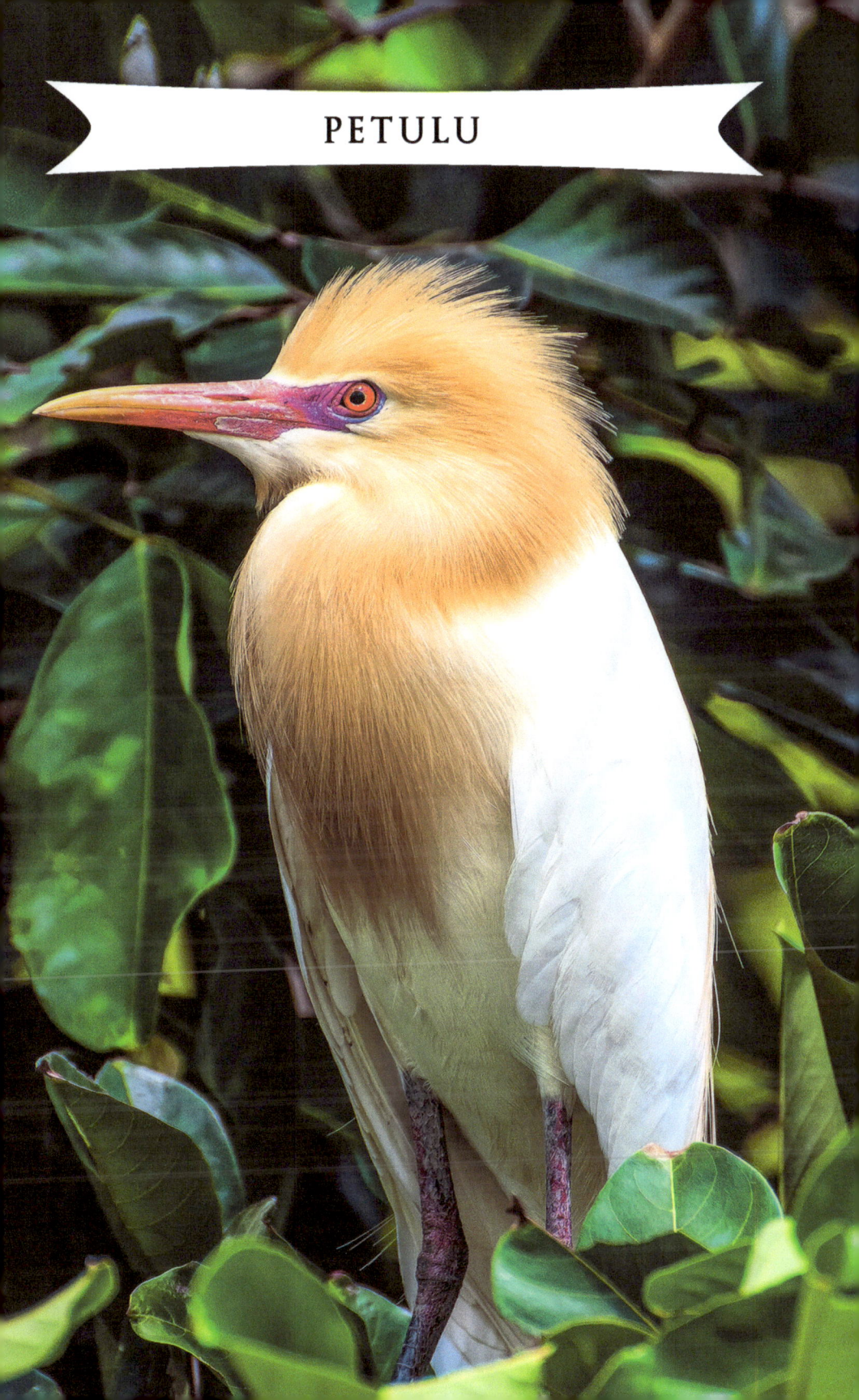

PETULU

PIGEON

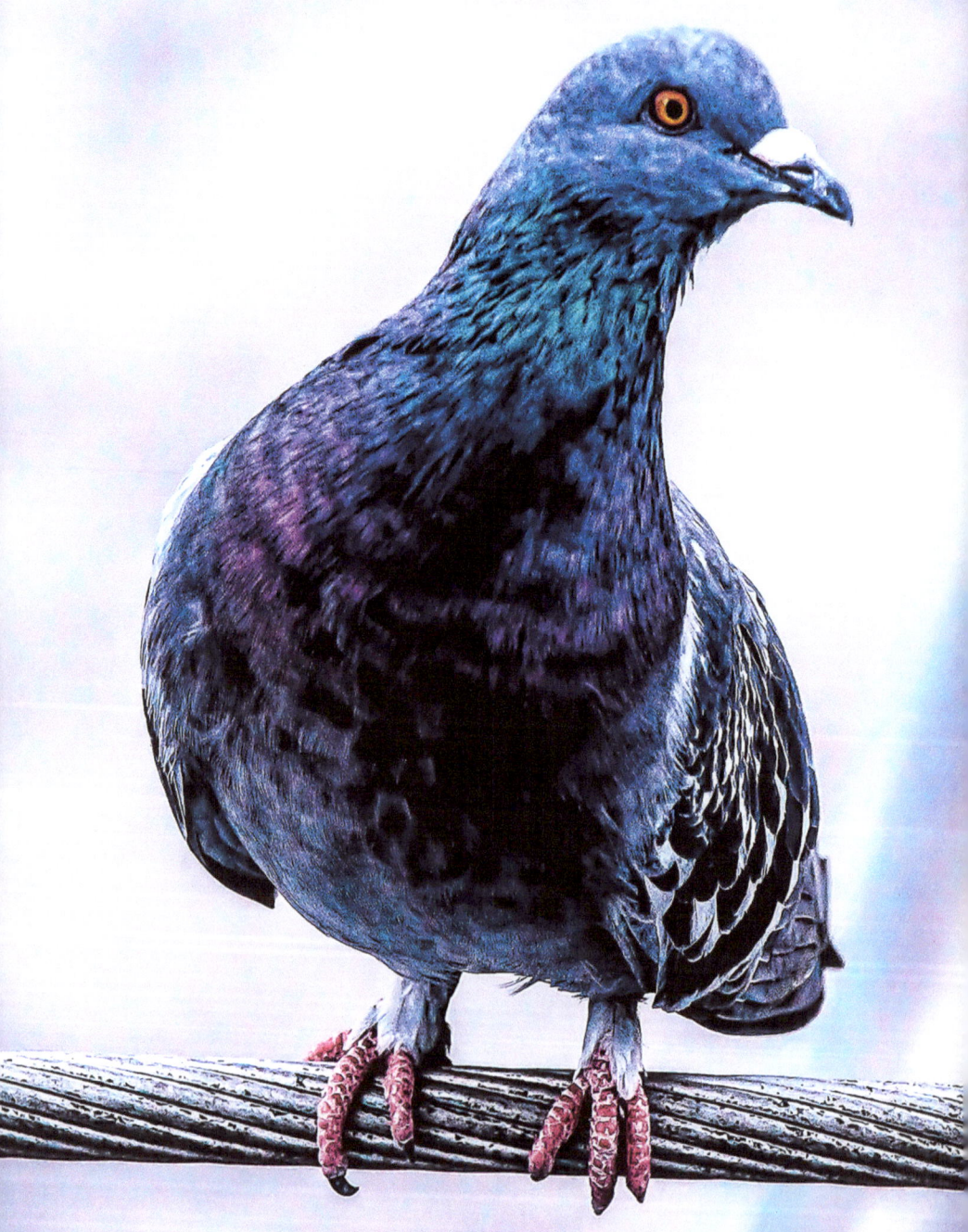

PHEASANT

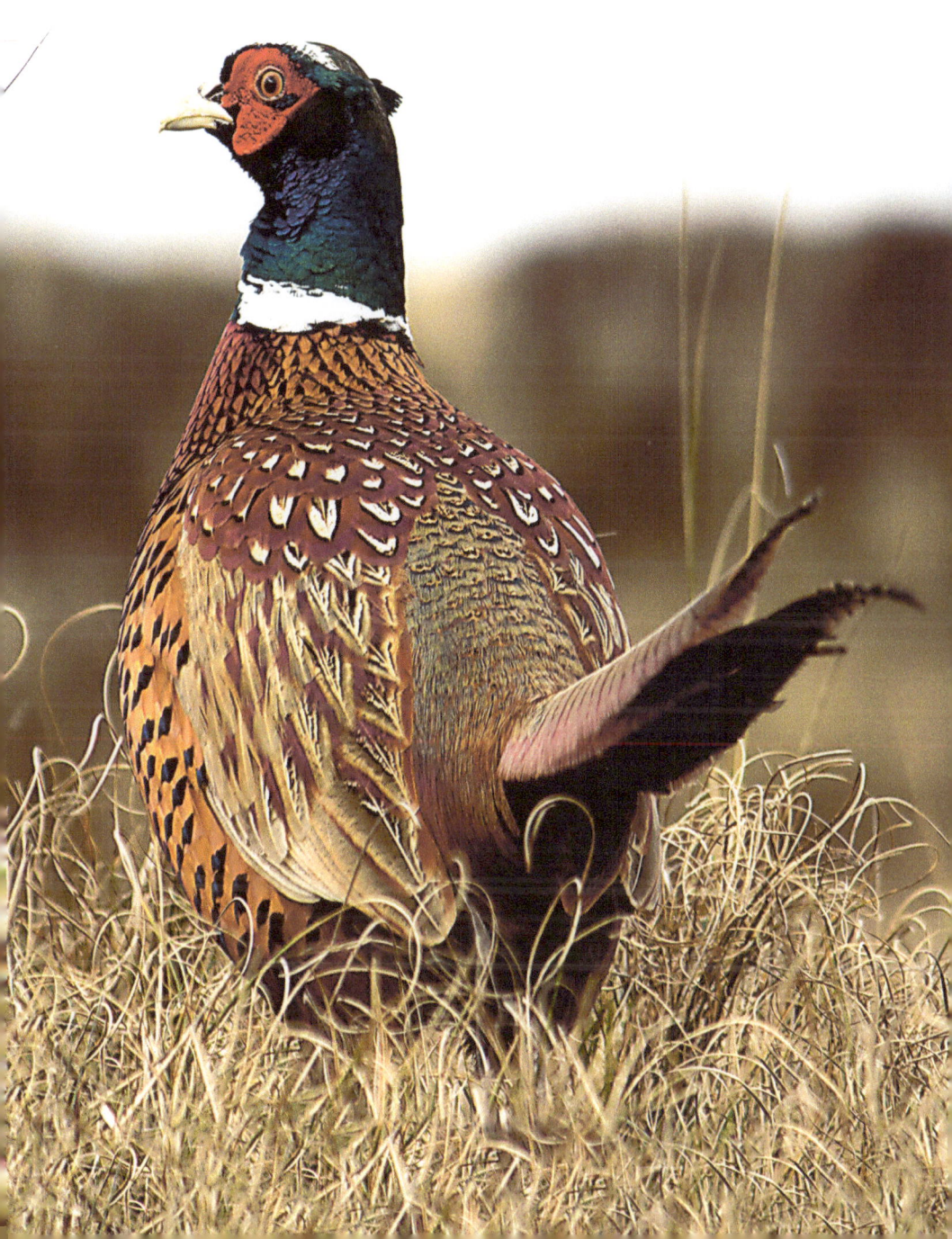

PURPLE FINCH

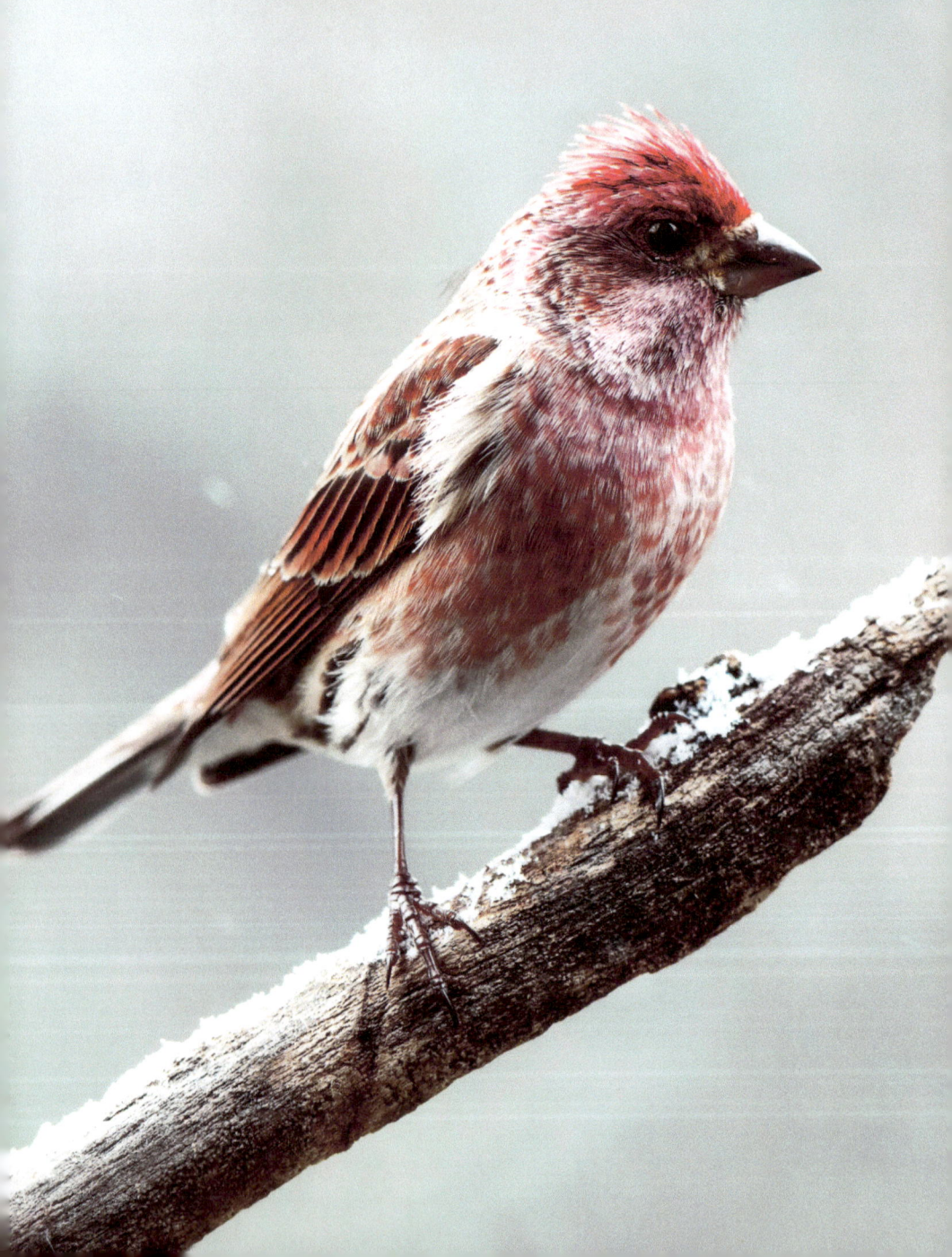

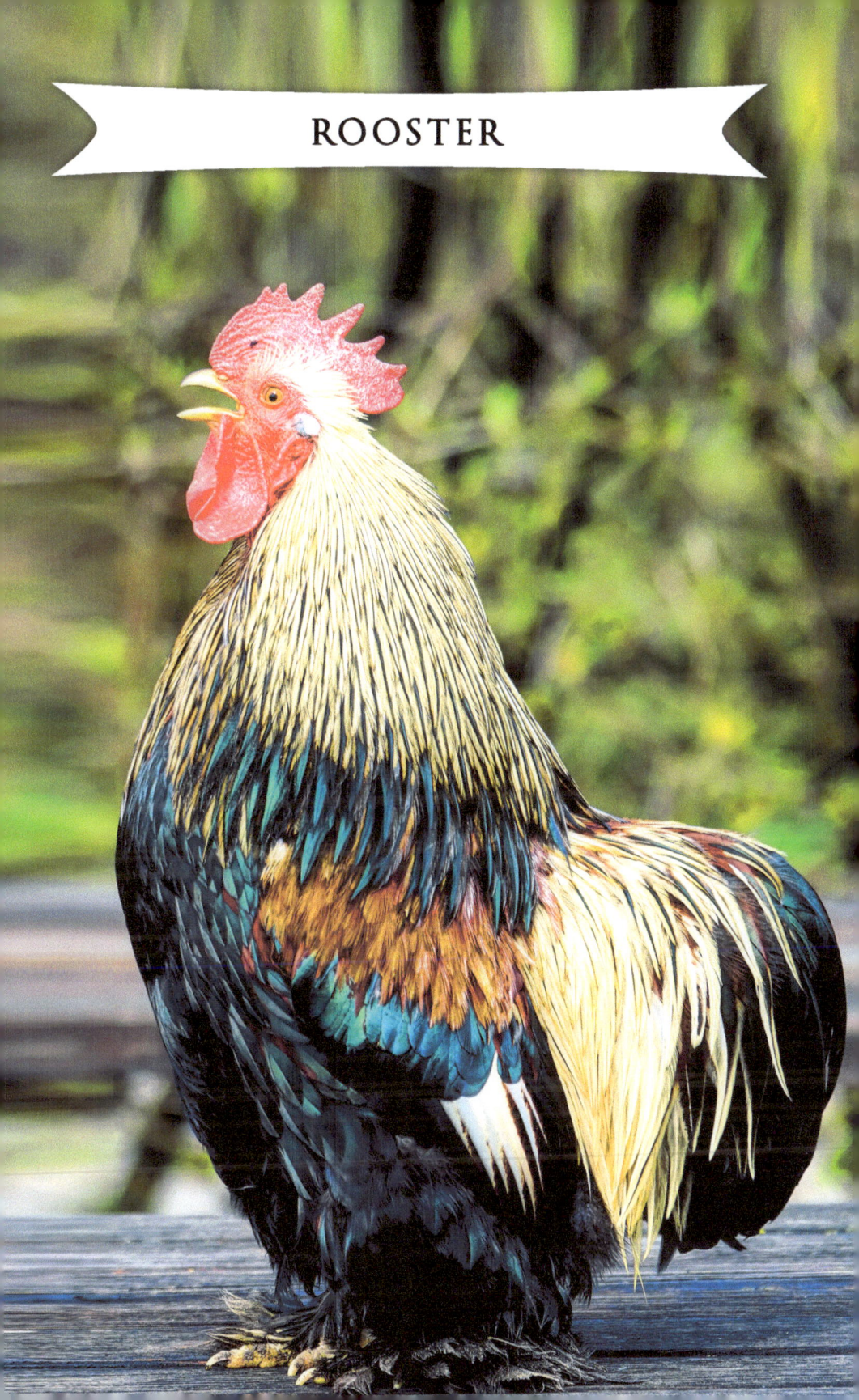

ROOSTER

SNOWY OWL

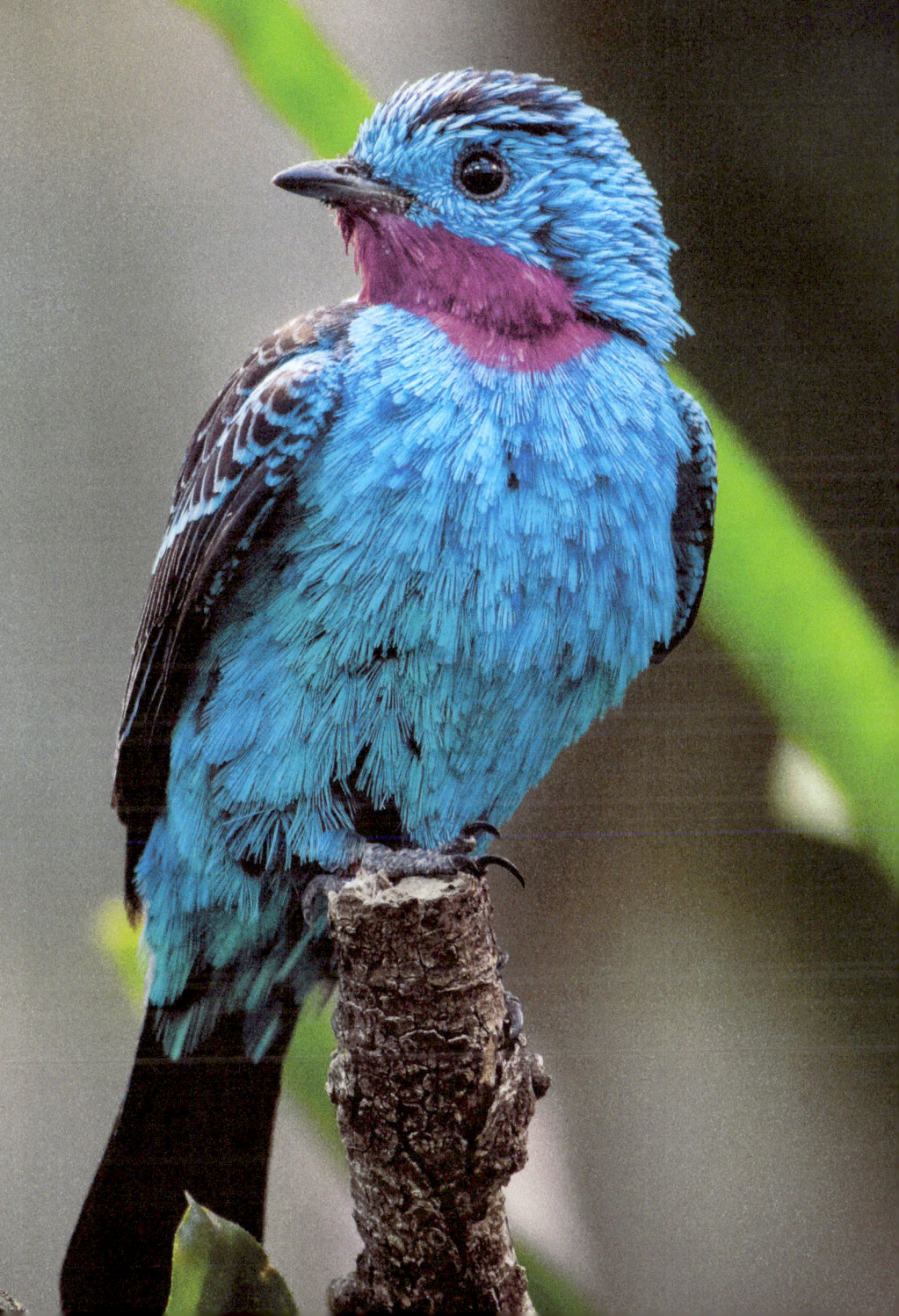

SPANGLED CONTINGA

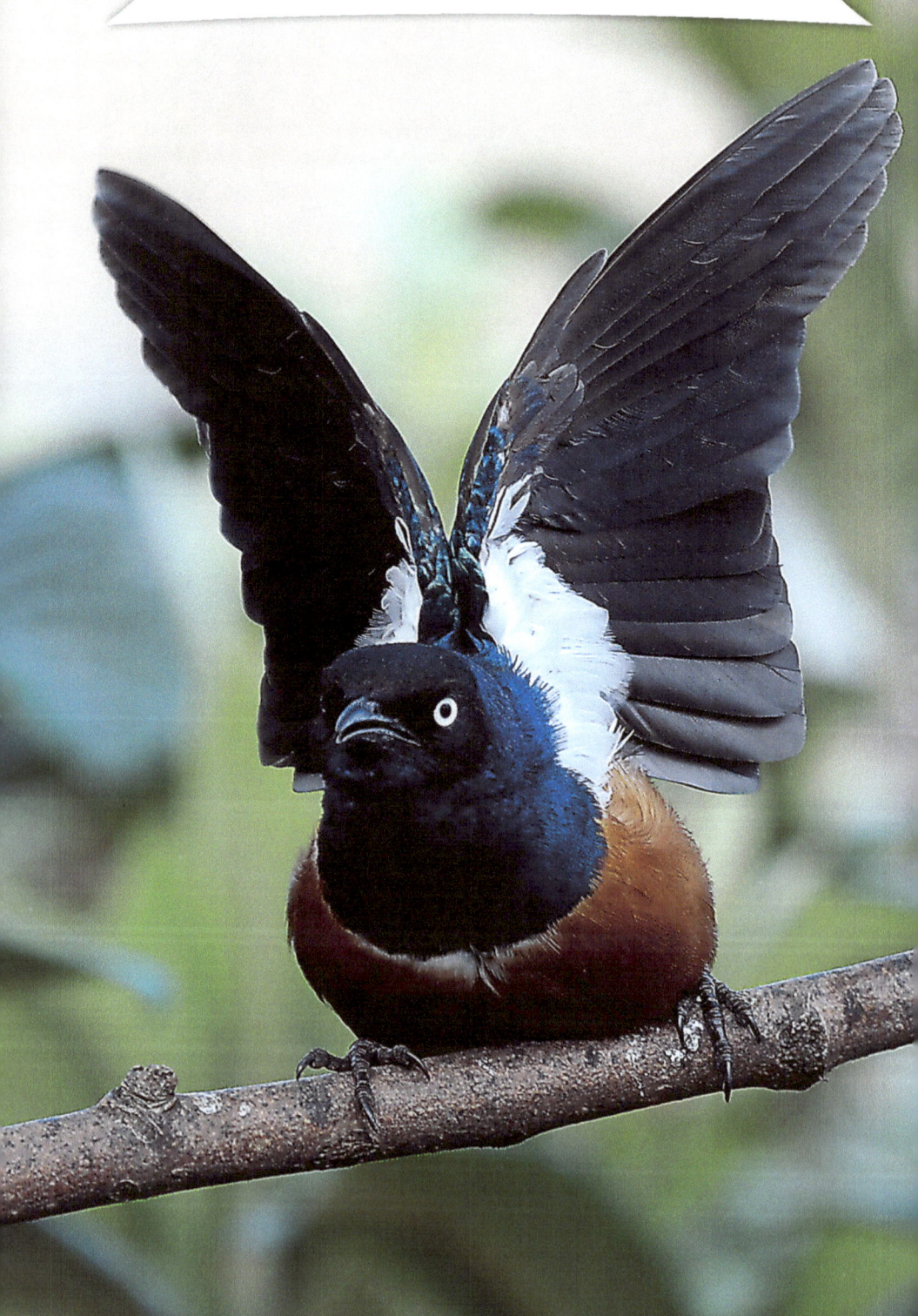

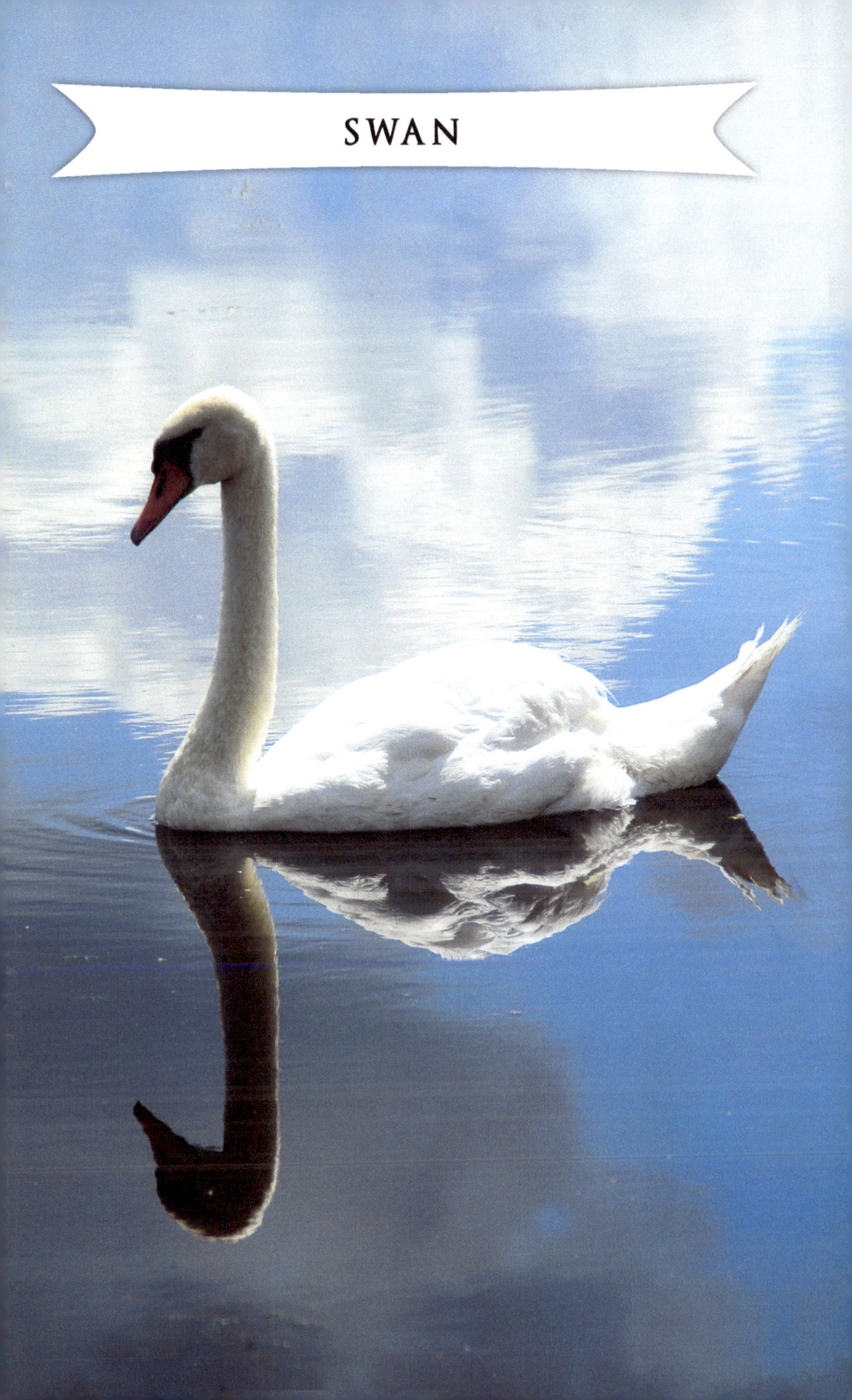

SWAN

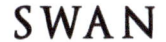

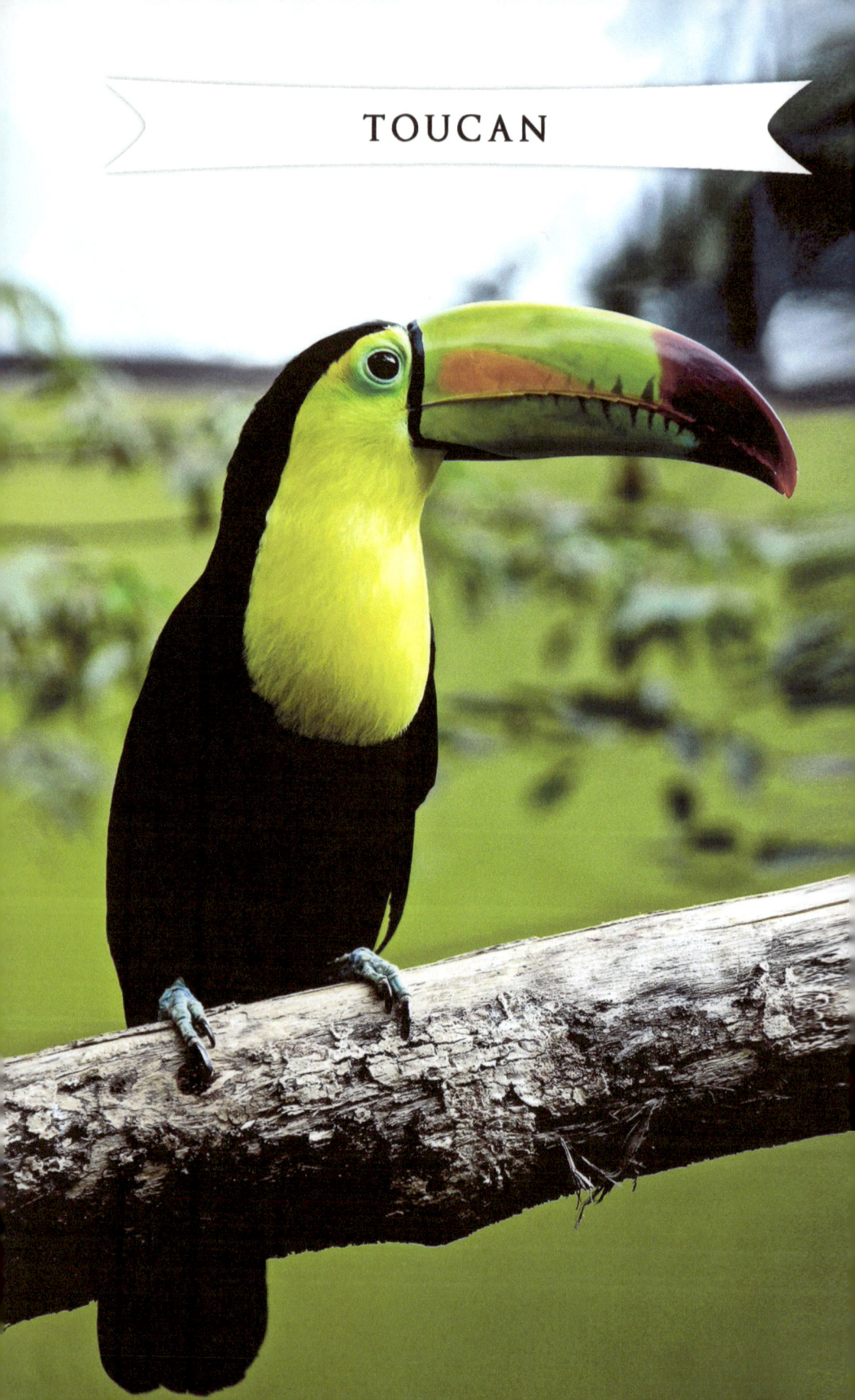

TOUCAN

WOODPECKER

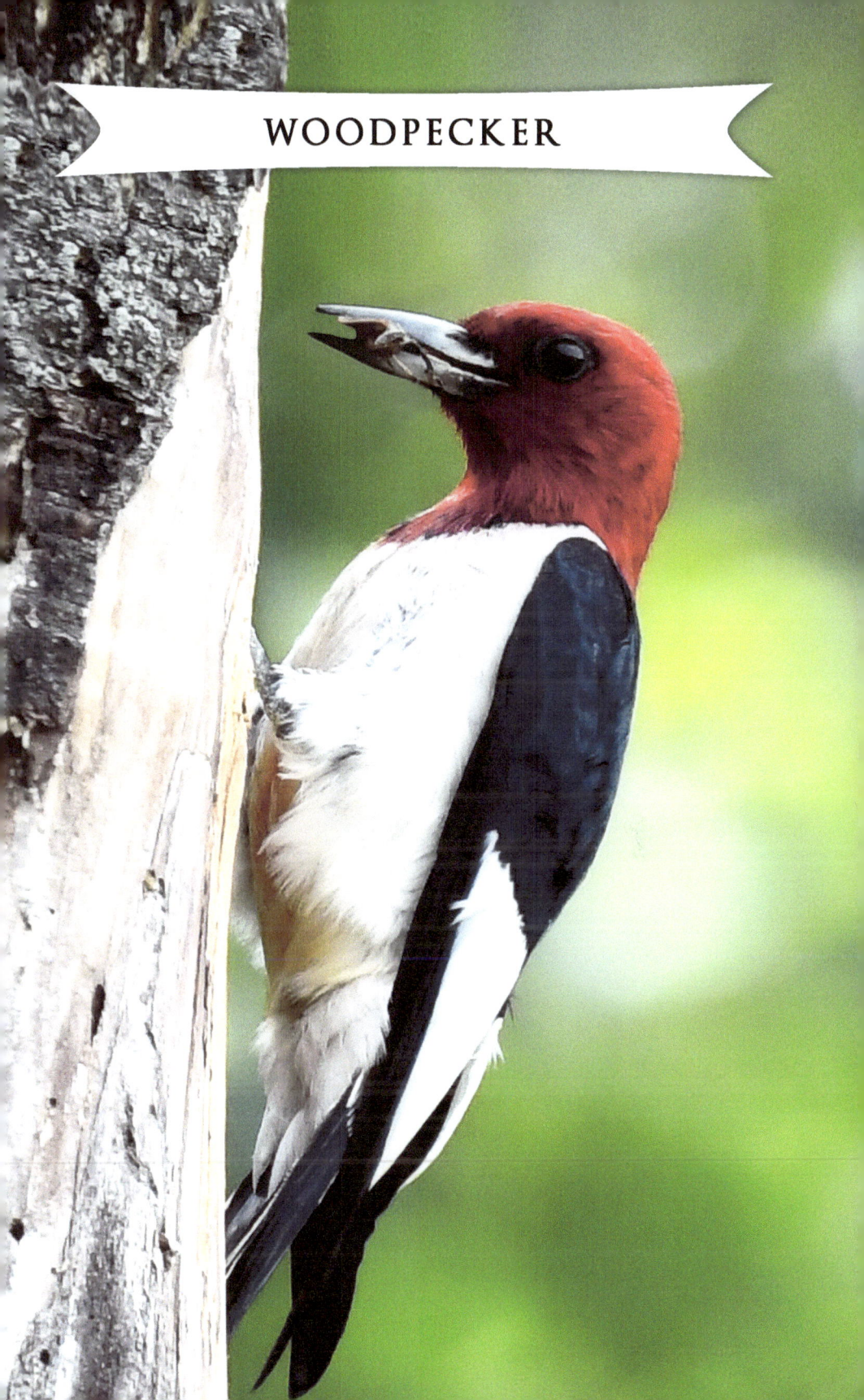

www.ingramcontent.com/pod-product-compliance
Lightning Source LLC
Chambersburg PA
CBHW050757290526
45792CB00008B/2215